"This is a great (and unique) bool[...]
diagnosis of borderline personality [...]
experts who study and treat BF[...]. [...] features of BPD are
described in very understandable terms, and there are clear suggestions for coping with these features and problems, as well as for
understanding their impact. I highly recommend this book for
those receiving the diagnosis, as well as for those with family
members or friends with BPD."

—**Timothy J. Trull, PhD**, curators' professor of
psychological sciences at the University of Missouri

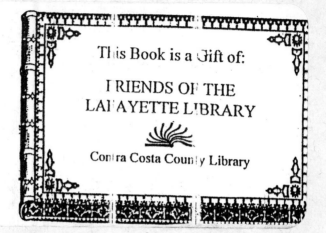

This Book is a Gift of:

FRIENDS OF THE
LAFAYETTE LIBRARY

Contra Costa County Library

GUIDES *for the* NEWLY DIAGNOSED
Series

New Harbinger's Newly Diagnosed book series was created to help people who have recently been diagnosed with a mental health condition. We understand that receiving a diagnosis can bring up many questions. For example, whom should you tell about your diagnosis? What treatments are available? What are the best techniques for managing your symptoms? And how do you start building a support network?

Our goal is to offer user-friendly resources that provide answers to these common questions, as well as evidence-based strategies to help you better cope with and manage your condition so you can get back to living a more balanced life.

Visit www.newharbinger.com for
more books in this series.

WITHDRAWN

Borderline Personality Disorder

A GUIDE *for* THE NEWLY DIAGNOSED

Alexander L. Chapman, PhD, RPsych
Kim L. Gratz, PhD

New Harbinger Publications, Inc.

Publisher's Note

This publication is designed to provide accurate and authoritative information in regard to the subject matter covered. It is sold with the understanding that the publisher is not engaged in rendering psychological, financial, legal, or other professional services. If expert assistance or counseling is needed, the services of a competent professional should be sought.

Distributed in Canada by Raincoast Books

Copyright © 2013 by Alexander L. Chapman and Kim L. Gratz
New Harbinger Publications, Inc.
5674 Shattuck Avenue
Oakland, CA 94609
www.newharbinger.com

Cover design by Amy Shoup
Acquired by Melissa Kirk
Edited by Jasmine Star

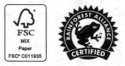

All Rights Reserved

Library of Congress Cataloging-in-Publication Data

Chapman, Alexander L. (Alexander Lawrence)
  Borderline personality disorder : a guide for the newly diagnosed / Alexander L.
Chapman, PhD, RPsych, and Kim L. Gratz, Gratz, PhD.
      pages cm -- (The new Harbinger guides for the newly diagnosed series)
  Summary: "Two experts on borderline personality disorder (BPD) present the fifth book
in the New Harbinger Guides for the Newly Diagnosed Series. This easy-to-read book
offers an introduction to BPD for those who have recently been diagnosed, outlines the
most common complications of the illness and the most effective treatments available, and
provides readers with practical strategies for staying on the path to recovery"-- Provided by
publisher.
  Includes bibliographical references.
  ISBN 978-1-60882-706-0 (pbk.) -- ISBN 978-1-60882-707-7 (pdf e-book) -- ISBN
978-1-60882-708-4 (ebook) 1. Borderline personality disorder. I. Gratz, Kim L. II. Title.
  RC569.5.B67C46 2013
  616.85'852--dc23

                                    2013023726

Printed in the United States of America

15   14   13

10   9   8   7   6   5   4   3   2   1   First printing

To those who suffer from BPD, I wish you freedom and joy.

—Alexander L. Chapman

To all those who struggle with BPD, I wish you self-compassion on your journey toward recovery.

—Kim L. Gratz

Contents

Acknowledgments

I'd like to acknowledge many people who have both supported my work on this book and helped me make it as useful as possible to those suffering from BPD. First, I've been fortunate enough to have wonderful mentors in my research work as well as in my clinical work, including Richard Farmer, Tony Cellucci, Thomas Lynch, Clive Robins, and Marsha Linehan. I am grateful for their guidance and wisdom. Second, I am so grateful to the clients with whom I have worked. Their courage in the face of overwhelming adversity is inspiring, and they have taught me more than I could have imagined about how to make my work and my writing as relevant as possible to what they struggle with each day. Finally, I'd like to express appreciation for my wonderfully supportive family.

—Alexander L. Chapman

I am extremely grateful to everyone who has traveled with me on this journey of helping those who suffer from BPD, including the mentors who trained me (Drs. Elizabeth Murphy, Liz Roemer, and John Gunderson), the clinicians who joined me on this path and devoted their time and energy to this lofty pursuit, and the clients who have graced me with their trust, courage, and commitment to recovery. I am also extraordinarily grateful to my DBT consultation team, particularly Katie Dixon-Gordon, for all that they do to help those who are suffering and to support one another through this process. I could not do this work without them. I am also incredibly thankful to have Daisy in my life, whose love and support makes everything better. Finally, as always, I am eternally grateful to Matt Tull and thankful to have him in my life. His love, friendship, encouragement, and support (both emotional and practical) make everything possible, and this book could not have been written without him.

—Kim L. Gratz

CHAPTER 1

⫸⫸⫸————————————————————⫷⫷⫷

YOU'VE BEEN DIAGNOSED WITH BORDERLINE PERSONALITY DISORDER: NOW WHAT?

If you are reading this book, chances are that you've recently been diagnosed with borderline personality disorder (BPD). If so, one question you may be asking yourself is *Now what?* That's a very good question. More often than not, books, websites, and even treatments for BPD don't pay much attention to the immediate aftermath of receiving a BPD diagnosis or how to handle the questions and emotions you may experience in response. Some of these resources may jump ahead and provide information on BPD, such as its causes or the types of problems that people with BPD may experience. Others may jump even further ahead to the skills you can use to manage the symptoms of BPD. As helpful as all of this information may be, however, it's okay to slow the process down.

Learning that you have BPD can be an emotional experience, both positive and negative, and you may not be ready to jump ahead just yet. The good news is that just learning that you have BPD and figuring out the next steps to take are crucial parts of the recovery process.

This chapter will lead you through some of the different things you can expect after learning that you meet criteria for a BPD diagnosis, as well as some of the first steps you can take once you receive this information.

DETERMINING IF THE DIAGNOSIS IS CORRECT

Being diagnosed with BPD can have a major impact on your life and the decisions you make about your mental health. Therefore, the first step after being diagnosed with BPD is to decide if you think the diagnosis is correct. To figure this out, you may want to consider who made the diagnosis and how it was made, and to ask any questions you may have about the diagnosis. It's also important to consider whether the diagnosis feels right to you. In the sections that follow, we'll take a closer look at each of these considerations.

Who Made the Diagnosis?

One of the first questions to ask yourself is whether a trained mental health professional gave you this diagnosis. These days, it's become increasingly common for people to turn to the Internet to try to diagnose themselves or their loved ones. When you or someone you love is struggling with a health problem (whether that problem is physical or mental), it's natural to try to get as much information as you can as quickly as possible. The Internet definitely takes the cake when it comes to having the most easily accessible information available on almost any topic you could imagine.

The problem with using the Internet to try to diagnose BPD is that the quality of the information that's available varies substantially. Some websites are excellent resources for learning more about BPD and provide detailed and accurate information on the symptoms of this disorder. In fact, we review some of these websites at the end of this chapter. Unfortunately, however, other websites provide inaccurate information on BPD or actually misrepresent what is known about this disorder. Attempts to diagnose someone based on this faulty information probably won't result in an accurate diagnosis.

In addition, trying to diagnose yourself with any disorder (physical or mental) is never recommended. It's common when reading about the symptoms of a disorder to begin to believe that you have those symptoms, even when you don't. In fact, this is such a common phenomenon in medical schools (where students must read about all kinds of disorders as part of their studies) that it's been given a name: medical student syndrome. Basically, the idea is that reading about symptoms can make people think they experience those symptoms far more often or intensely than they actually do. Therefore, attempting to diagnose yourself with BPD probably won't work either. The bottom line is that your best bet for getting an accurate diagnosis is to meet with a trained mental health professional.

How Was the Diagnosis Made?

Determining whether a person has BPD is not a simple process. Therefore, it's important to know how your clinician arrived at the diagnosis and the steps she or he took to get there. Only then will you know whether the diagnosis seems sound.

Within the mental health profession, the gold standard for determining mental health diagnoses is a *structured clinical interview*. In a structured clinical interview, the clinician will ask you a specific set of questions about your mood and behaviors. For example, to see whether you have symptoms of BPD, the clinician may ask, "Do you often experience shifts in your mood?" or "Have you had relationships characterized by frequent arguments or breakups?" The clinician may also ask you to elaborate on certain answers or give specific examples of what you're talking about. Don't hesitate to provide as much information as you can. Also, it's important to be as honest as you can during the interview. Clinicians can base a diagnosis only on what clients tell them.

In addition to asking you questions about the symptoms of BPD, many clinicians will ask you about past experiences, your family history, and symptoms of other disorders. This is done to make sure that the symptoms you describe are best explained by

BPD and not some other diagnosis, such as a mood disorder, post-traumatic stress disorder, or a physical health condition. Once the interview is complete, the clinician will review your responses and determine whether you experience enough symptoms to qualify for a diagnosis of BPD. Currently, out of the nine symptoms of BPD (which we will discuss in detail in chapter 2), you need to experience only five to meet criteria for BPD (American Psychiatric Association 2000).

Some clinicians may not use a structured clinical interview to diagnose BPD. Although this is the gold standard, there are other ways of determining whether someone qualifies for a BPD diagnosis. For example, some clinicians may have you complete a questionnaire that asks about a number of different symptoms you may be experiencing. A benefit of this approach is that it's usually much quicker than a structured interview, so you may be able to receive a diagnosis in a shorter period of time. However, using questionnaires alone to diagnose BPD has some downsides. In particular, because questionnaires require you to choose the best option from a limited number of choices, they don't allow clinicians to get a complete understanding of when, how often, and in what type of situations you experience specific symptoms. Therefore, questionnaires alone are unlikely to provide the detailed information needed to arrive at an accurate diagnosis of BPD.

If your clinician based your BPD diagnosis solely on your answers to one or more questionnaires, there's a good chance that she or he may not have had all the information needed to reach an accurate diagnosis. That said, some questionnaires have been shown to do a good job of identifying people who struggle with

BPD symptoms, and these may be a useful first step in a clinician's efforts to determine whether you have BPD. However, regardless of how helpful a questionnaire may be, we believe that it is only a first step in figuring out whether someone has BPD and a starting point for a larger discussion with a clinician about one's symptoms.

Be Sure to Ask Questions Yourself

Once a clinician gives you a BPD diagnosis, it's your turn to ask the questions. In the process of giving someone a diagnosis, many clinicians explain how they reached their decision and the different factors they took into consideration. If your clinician doesn't give you this information up front, don't be afraid to ask for it. In fact, no matter how much information the clinician provides, don't hesitate to ask as many questions as you want. That's how you'll know whether the diagnosis seems right to you.

If you're not sure what types of questions to ask, here are some that may be useful. First, if the clinician hasn't already answered this question to your satisfaction, you may want to ask why she or he thinks you have BPD and the specific information that led to this conclusion. This should be easy enough for any clinician to answer and can give you a much better idea about how the diagnosis fits you personally. Along these same lines, it's also important to ask which specific symptoms of BPD you have. For example, you might ask the clinician to review each of the BPD symptoms with you and explain what it takes to meet criteria for each. Finally, you may also want to make sure that the clinician considered other diagnoses, in addition to or instead of

BPD. You may want to ask whether the clinician collected information on other disorders you may have and, if so, what those disorders were and why BPD was selected instead of (or in addition to) the others.

Does the Diagnosis Feel Right?

It's also important to ask yourself whether the diagnosis of BPD seems to fit with your experience. Take some time to review the symptoms of BPD and think about whether they seem to apply to you. Do the symptoms fit with what you've experienced? Does the diagnosis help you organize or better understand the various thoughts, behaviors, and emotions you've been struggling with? Does the diagnosis make sense to you? Trust your gut reaction. If it seems like the symptoms don't describe your experiences or the problems you're struggling with, talk with the clinician about doing a more thorough assessment or considering other possibilities. In the end, your diagnosis is going to guide your treatment options and the decisions you make on the road to recovery. Therefore, you want to make sure that it truly represents your behaviors, thoughts, and emotions.

Get a Second Opinion

So, what happens if you talk with the clinician about your diagnosis, ask all of the questions you have, and read over the symptoms of BPD on your own and still feel like the diagnosis doesn't seem right? In that case, it's completely reasonable to get a second opinion. Many people get second opinions after receiving a diagnosis of a physical illness or disease. Getting a diagnosis from a mental health professional is no different. Reaching a diagnosis is not a perfect science. Errors can be made, and different people may have different opinions. If you have any reason to doubt the clinician's decision, or if you just want the additional comfort of knowing that no stone was left unturned in determining whether you have BPD, seek the assistance of another clinician and have that person conduct a separate assessment.

MANAGING EMOTIONAL REACTIONS TO YOUR DIAGNOSIS

Receiving a BPD diagnosis can lead to a number of different emotions and thoughts. For some people, it can provide a sense of relief. Many people with BPD struggle with their symptoms for years before they are diagnosed, not knowing why they're struggling or how to make sense of their difficulties. Therefore, just knowing that these symptoms have a name and are shared by a number of other people can be quite a relief.

Think about your experience before you were diagnosed with BPD. Prior to receiving the diagnosis, you might have felt as though something was wrong with you or that you were different from everyone else. You might have wondered why your feelings and relationships seemed so much more challenging than those of other people or why you struggled so much of the time. You may have felt alone in your experiences, like you were an alien or the proverbial black sheep. The combination of not knowing why you're struggling and feeling alone in that struggle can be a difficult and painful experience. It can make you question your thoughts, emotions, and everyday experiences. It can contribute to feelings of helplessness and hopelessness. It can make you doubt yourself.

Therefore, receiving a diagnosis of BPD—learning that there is actually a name for the set of symptoms you've been experiencing—may provide some relief. Getting a diagnosis can provide you with a way of understanding and making sense of your experiences and help you feel less alone. Learning that the symptoms you've been struggling with are common enough to have been included in the diagnostic manual for mental disorders shows you that other people also experience these symptoms. It also indicates that researchers and clinicians are aware of BPD and are striving to learn more about it and how best to treat it. All of this can contribute to a sense of relief. Knowing what you have is the first step in addressing it. Learning that you have BPD means that you can now take steps to overcome it. You may feel more hopeful about the future and less helpless about how to address your symptoms.

That said, we don't mean to imply that it's easy to receive a BPD diagnosis or that you won't also experience feelings of fear, anger, sadness, or shame in response. These are all very understandable reactions. When you consider how much misinformation there is about BPD, it's easy to see how someone could have negative beliefs or misconceptions about being diagnosed with BPD. Although these beliefs definitely aren't accurate and can easily be changed just by learning more about this disorder, it's understandable that they could lead to feelings of sadness or shame as a result of learning that you have BPD.

Other common reactions to receiving a BPD diagnosis are fear and anxiety. Being diagnosed with BPD can be an overwhelming experience. You may not know what to expect or the next steps to take. You may understand that you need to get help but not know what treatment options are available or which is the best treatment. You may also wonder whether, when, or how to tell other people about your diagnosis. As a result, it would make a lot of sense if you experienced anxiety, fear, or worries about the future.

Finally, some people feel as though their lives are already out of control and the diagnosis of BPD is just one more weight that they have to carry. They may also start to think about the negative experiences they have had, such as abuse or neglect, that may have led to some of the symptoms of BPD. This could lead to feelings of anger about having a BPD diagnosis.

Regardless of what emotions you experience, positive or negative, being diagnosed with BPD can be an intense and overwhelming experience. For this reason, it can be helpful to learn some basic coping strategies to manage any emotions you may experience. In the sections that follow, we'll review some strategies you might find helpful soon after receiving a BPD diagnosis. We will discuss some of these strategies, as well as other coping skills for managing distressing emotions, in detail later in the book. For now, though, the strategies outlined below may be a useful first step in coping with some of the emotions you may experience upon learning your diagnosis.

Don't Do Anything (at First)

Although not doing anything might sound like a strange suggestion, it's important to give yourself some time to let your new diagnosis sink in. Resist the urge to make any immediate decisions or changes in your life. Instead, now more than ever, it's important to have some stability in your life. One way to do this is to maintain your daily schedule: waking up around the same time every morning, going to school or work as usual, and spending time with the people you care about. After being diagnosed with BPD, some people feel as if life has been turned upside down. By maintaining a set schedule and continuing to do the day-to-day activities you've always done, you can maintain some sense of predictability and certainty in your life. This will also help you establish a sense of control over your life, which can be particularly important if things feel chaotic and stressful.

Seek Support

It may also be helpful to seek support from people you trust and in whom you have confided in the past. Now, whether you feel comfortable sharing your diagnosis with others is something only you can decide. There is definitely no need to tell others, particularly before you've processed the news yourself. That said, some people find it helpful to talk through the diagnosis and their reactions to it with friends or family. If you choose to do this, it may be helpful to share the symptoms associated with BPD, as well as information on how it develops and is diagnosed and treated. They may have a lot of questions (just as you likely do), and it can be helpful to seek the answers together.

Practice Self-Care

Practicing self-care will be especially important if you are experiencing feelings of shame, anger, fear, or sadness. Approach yourself with compassion. Receiving a diagnosis of BPD can be stressful. Therefore, it's very important to schedule comforting, pleasant, and relaxing activities during your day. Soak in a warm bath. Eat a comforting meal. Go see a funny movie or watch your favorite television show. Light a scented candle or drink a warm cup of herbal tea. All of these activities can help take the edge off of intense, unpleasant emotions and may give you some relief.

It can also be helpful to spend some time brainstorming specific things you can do when certain emotions, such as shame or anger, are really intense. Making a list ahead of time of things you can do when you feel intense emotions can make it easier to resist urges to do things you might later regret. Remember, regardless of how you feel on the inside or what your thoughts are telling you, you are in control of your behaviors. Choosing to do something healthy rather than acting on the urges that go along with shame or anger can be a useful way of managing those feelings and preventing them from sticking around longer than necessary or becoming more intense.

Acknowledge and Respect Your Emotions

Regardless of the particular emotions you experience in response to receiving a diagnosis of BPD, they are there for a reason. They make sense. As we discussed above, there are many reasons you might experience anger, sadness, fear, or even relief. Some of these emotions may feel unpleasant; however, it's important to make room for them and not push them away. Emotions serve an important function in people's lives. They are the body's way of communicating with us. They provide us with information.

Anger may tell us that we've been violated in some way or feel as though things are out of control. Anxiety and fear can tell us that we're experiencing a threat to our well-being. Sadness tells us that we're experiencing a loss. Listen to the information your emotions are providing you. The more you attend to your emotions, the less likely they are to become intense or hang around for a long time. Try to understand why you're experiencing a certain emotion, and give yourself permission to have that emotion and to express it. Take the time to feel and work through the emotions you're having as a result of learning that you have BPD.

Seek Information

Finally, an excellent way of coping with the stress associated with receiving a diagnosis of BPD is to seek as much information as you can about BPD. If you were just diagnosed with BPD, you may be asking yourself questions like *Why me?* or *Why do I have this symptom and not others?* You may also wonder what treatments are available for BPD and how helpful these treatments are. Simply learning more about BPD can be a useful way to alleviate some of the anxiety, shame, and other emotions that may arise from these kinds of questions.

So, where do you find good information on BPD? Well, if you're reading this book, that's definitely a start. Keep reading! This book will provide a wealth of information on BPD. You may also be inclined to check out the Internet for information. As we mentioned above, the Internet can be an excellent source of information, but you need to be careful; there's a lot of misinformation about BPD on the web. Therefore, we recommend that you use caution when turning to the Internet for information. To help you separate the wheat from the chaff, here are some websites that provide good, up-to-date, and accurate information on BPD:

- National Education Alliance for BPD (NEA.BPD): www.borderlinepersonalitydisorder.com

- Treatment and Research Advancements National Association for Personality Disorder (TARA NAPD): www.tara4bpd.org

- National Institute of Mental Health (NIMH): www.nimh.nih.gov/health/topics/ borderline-personality-disorder

- American Psychological Association (APA): www.apa.org/topics/personality

- National Alliance on Mental Illness (NAMI): www.nami.org

- BPD Central: www.bpdcentral.com

- Behavioral Tech, LLC: www.behavioraltech.org

This is by no means an exhaustive list of good Internet resources on BPD; however, it is a good place to start. It may also be worthwhile to talk with your clinician or other mental health professionals in your area to see if they can recommend any resources.

MOVING FORWARD

Now that you've read this chapter, you're well on your way toward overcoming BPD. We hope that you've already learned some facts about BPD that you didn't know before. We also hope that you feel more confident and clear about how you can move forward. If not, that's okay. This is a process, and we'll be right there with you along the way.

The next few chapters in this book provide information on the symptoms of BPD, how it develops, and treatments that work. Later chapters will help you learn healthy coping skills for managing your symptoms. We hope that you'll gain additional clarity and insight into BPD with each chapter you read, and that this insight will help you feel more empowered and hopeful about your future. Let's get started!

CHAPTER 2

WHAT IS BPD?

Julie left her appointment with Dr. Jones, a psychologist, with her head spinning, feeling both relieved and anxious. Ever since her early teens, Julie knew that there was something different about her. She was like a walking emotional barometer, noticing very quickly when other people around her were upset. She went through periods when she experienced seemingly inexplicable, unbearable emotional pain that nobody seemed to understand. At these times, only cutting herself and drinking alcohol seemed to lighten the load and give her some relief. Although she knew it wasn't necessarily rational, she often got swept up in fears that her close friends or partners were going to leave her alone, without anyone to support her. She had been to several therapists but kept getting conflicting information. Some told her she might be developing bipolar disorder, and others said she had an anxiety disorder or depression. When she looked up these diagnoses, they didn't really seem to fit, so she did some research on her own, talked to her psychiatrist, and got a referral to a psychologist with a specialty in personality disorders. When Dr. Jones told her that she had borderline personality disorder and explained what this meant, Julie felt relieved that there was finally a name for her problems, with a description that really seemed to fit. At the same time, she felt overwhelmed about what to do next and anxious about the road to recovery ahead.

It's very important that you know exactly what your diagnosis of BPD means. We've worked with a number of clients who had been recently diagnosed with BPD and showed up at our clinics feeling confused, overwhelmed, and surprised. Such clients often don't have a clear idea of what BPD actually is or what to do next. Although receiving a diagnosis of BPD is one of the first steps on the road to recovery, it will be helpful only if you know what the diagnosis means. In this chapter, we'll shed some light on exactly what you're dealing with if you've been diagnosed with BPD.

PERSONALITY DISORDERS

Let's start by talking a bit about personality disorders in general. When we talk about someone's personality, we're talking about that person's typical ways of acting, feeling, thinking, and relating to the world. A *personality disorder* is a long-standing pattern of relating to the world that doesn't work very well and causes problems or distress for people. There are many different types of personality disorders, including obsessive-compulsive, dependent, paranoid, narcissistic, antisocial, and of course, BPD. "Personality disorder" isn't actually the most useful or descriptive term. It suggests a lot of things that just aren't true, such as that there's something wrong with the person's personality, that the problems are all in the person's head, or that this will be a lifelong problem. As you'll learn in this chapter and the next three, none of these things are true, and there is actually a lot of hope for people who have been diagnosed with BPD.

BORDERLINE PERSONALITY DISORDER

BPD is a disorder involving instability in many areas of life, including emotions, relationships, behavior, and identity. As mentioned, to be diagnosed with BPD, you must have at least five of nine key symptoms (American Psychiatric Association 2000):

- Persistent and strong efforts to avoid real or imagined abandonment by others

- A pattern of unstable, intense, and stormy relationships where you may shift between idealizing and devaluing your partner

- Lack of a cohesive identity or a poor or unstable self-image or sense of self

- Impulsive and self-destructive behaviors, such as substance use, sexual promiscuity, reckless driving, or binge eating

- Reoccurring acts of suicidal behavior, threats of suicide, or deliberate self-harm, such as cutting or burning yourself

- Frequent and intense mood swings

- Chronic feelings of emptiness

- The intense experience of anger, difficulties controlling anger, or both

- Paranoia or dissociation that comes and goes as a result of experiencing stress

In the sections that follow, we'll take a closer look at these symptoms. Ultimately, most of them boil down to instability in four key areas: emotions, relationships, behavior, and identity.

Unstable Emotions

If you have BPD, you might feel like you're on an emotional roller-coaster ride, at times feeling joyful and then, at the drop of a hat, feeling intense negative emotions. It might seem as though there's no rhyme or reason to your emotions, and you may feel demoralized and confused much of the time. Emotions that are particularly tough for people with BPD include sadness, shame, loneliness, fear, and anger toward themselves.

Perhaps you've struggled with these emotions as well. While this is challenging, there is a positive side to being highly emotional: you may experience life more fully, be more sensitive and passionate than other people, and be more attuned to others' feelings. However, if you're highly emotional and don't know how to manage your emotions, it may feel as though your life is spinning out of control, and your emotions can start to seem uncontrollable and even unbearable.

Unstable Relationships

Your relationships might follow a roller-coaster pattern similar to that of your emotions. When things go really well with your friends, partners, or family members, you might feel wonderful— supported and cared for. But when conflict arises, it might seem as though the relationship is fraught with misery, chaos, and rejection. Indeed, people with BPD often fear rejection and abandonment. They're quick to hear the alarm bells that someone might be leaving them (even when it's a false alarm) and sometimes go to great lengths to prevent relationships from ending. Some people with BPD alternate between intense love and hatred toward the people they're closest to and may experience so much anger that they feel like they could explode. Others are very sensitive to others' tone of voice and demeanor and may feel particularly devastated or alone if they sense irritation, emotional withdrawal, or a lack of support from others.

If you have BPD, you may have experienced some or all of these symptoms. Perhaps you've also felt guilty or ashamed about things you have done or said in the midst of relationship storms. The flip side is that people with BPD are often particularly attentive to relationships. You might pay a lot of attention to other people and be very attuned to how they're feeling. You probably care deeply about others, and your relationships are probably very important to you. However, for reasons we describe below, people with BPD have great difficulty navigating the often uncertain and rocky terrain of close relationships.

Unstable Behavior

Another area of instability that goes along with BPD is in regard to behavior. Have you ever found yourself doing reckless things without thinking about the consequences? Have you done things you later regretted in an attempt to escape emotional pain in the moment? Some common behaviors that go along with BPD include drinking excessively, using recreational drugs, engaging in risky sexual encounters, spending impulsively, binge eating, and driving recklessly. People with BPD often engage in these types of behaviors impulsively, without thinking of the longer-term consequences. Other examples include self-harm and suicide attempts. In fact, up to 80 percent of people with BPD report engaging in self-harming behaviors (Lieb et al. 2004), and up to 75 percent report having attempted suicide at some point in their lives (Frances, Fyer, and Clarkin 1986). Most people with BPD harm themselves or attempt suicide to escape emotional pain (Chapman, Gratz, and Brown 2006).

If you have BPD, you might have a hard time stopping yourself from acting on urges to do some of the things we described above. Impulsivity is common among people with BPD and is one of the key personality traits underlying BPD (American Psychiatric Association 2000). Being an impulsive person can make you spontaneous, fun, and willing to take risks, exposing you to new experiences that you might have shied away from if you were more fearful or inhibited. But as you can see, there's also a dark side to impulsivity, and it can lead to immense pain and suffering.

Unstable Identity

People with BPD often have an unstable sense of identity. From what you've read about BPD so far, this probably makes a lot of sense. If your emotions and relationships are unstable and out of control, and if you see yourself doing things that aren't in your long-term best interest, you might have a hard time figuring out who the "real you" actually is. Some people think we form a consistent sense of identity by reflecting on our history, what we've done and been through, our likes and dislikes, our hobbies and interests, our values, our relationships, and other qualities that make us who we are. This is like having a story, or narrative, that helps you answer the question of who you are. If you think about a character from a fairy tale, for example, Snow White, you probably have a consistent thread or story in your mind about her history, what she's generally like as a person, and what she's likely to do in certain circumstances (particularly when Prince Charming shows up!).

But if you can't trust your own brain, don't understand (and can't stand) your emotions, have tumultuous relationships, and have trouble remembering specific facts or events in your history (as people with BPD sometimes do), it can be hard to maintain a clear sense of who you are. It's like trying to shoot an arrow at a moving target. If you have BPD, you might be able to relate to this sense of an unclear identity. And for many people with BPD, this trait goes hand in hand with a persistent, painful feeling of emptiness and a sense that they are nobody or don't even exist. In fact, this can be the reason it's so hard when relationships end. People with BPD may define themselves by who they are in a relationship with. Therefore, if a key relationship ends, they might feel as if they're dropping into an abyss and losing their sense of who they are.

BPD IS NOT A DISEASE

Now that we've explained the symptoms characteristic of BPD, there are a few more important things for you to know. First, BPD is a collection of emotions, thoughts, and actions that probably cause you distress and create problems in your life. We don't believe that BPD is a disease. In fact, there's a lot of evidence that the core traits of BPD, such as emotional vulnerability and impulsivity, exist within a lot of people to some degree. Therefore, it's more accurate to think of BPD as a disorder with varying degrees of severity, rather than as a disorder that you either have or don't have. Also, there's no evidence that some kind of disease process, infection, virus, or environmental pathogen or toxin causes BPD, nor is BPD caused by poor diet or unhealthful lifestyle choices. Therefore, we don't think of BPD in the same way as we would a medical disease, such as diabetes or cancer.

Second, knowing you have BPD doesn't tell you (or anyone else, for that matter) exactly who you are or what you're like, just as knowing that something is a cake doesn't tell you exactly what it's made of or how it will taste. The specific ingredients matter.

CAUSES OF BPD

If you were diagnosed with BPD recently, you're probably wondering how you ended up with BPD in the first place. After decades of research, all that can be said with certainty is that researchers aren't entirely sure what causes BPD, and that the causes are probably different for different people. This is probably not the most reassuring, satisfying answer, but it's true. However, we can give you a good sense of the factors that probably work together to cause BPD. As you read through the following sections, please keep in mind that mental health problems as complex as BPD are rarely, if ever, caused by one thing alone.

Genes and BPD

You may wonder whether you can inherit BPD. To some extent, BPD does run in families. For instance, a few studies have shown that between 10 and 20 percent of parents and siblings of people with BPD also have BPD (Zanarini et al. 1988). Although 10 to 20 percent may not sound high, consider that 20 percent is nearly ten times higher than the prevalence of BPD in the general community. Also, studies indicate that identical twins are more likely to both have BPD than are fraternal twins (Torgersen 2000). Because identical twins share 100 percent of their genes whereas fraternal twins share only about 50 percent, this suggests that something genetic is involved in the development of BPD.

Overall, scientists have estimated that BPD is about 50 percent heritable, meaning that, in the general population, about half of the cases of BPD can be attributed to genetic factors. This doesn't mean 50 percent of BPD for any specific person is due to genes and the other 50 percent is due to other factors, nor does it mean that BPD is 100 percent genetic for some people and 0 percent genetic for others. Heritability only says something about how well we can predict who in a large group of people might have BPD, not what caused BPD for any individual in that group. Moreover, we know that it's likely that many genes working together influence the development of BPD, not a single gene operating all alone. Furthermore, we think different combinations of genetic, biological, neurological, and environmental factors cause BPD in different people.

BPD, Temperament, and the Brain

This brings us to the brain. Given that the genetic blueprints for your body and brain have some differences from those of other people, this could certainly result in differences in your brain. As mentioned, people with BPD often are very emotionally sensitive, reacting to things that may not phase other people; have stronger emotional reactions than others do; and take a long time to return to a calm, even emotional state after getting upset (Linehan

1993a). We think of this as having a very emotional temperament. You might wonder where would you get such an emotional temperament. As with most of the things that make us who we are, this probably arises due to a combination of your biology and brain and your environment and experiences.

In terms of the brain, it's important to know that certain brain areas are involved in how emotional you are and how strongly you react to stress. Research shows that at least two brain systems are different in people with BPD compared with those who don't have BPD. For example, the amygdala, an area of the brain thought of as its "emotional engine" (because it's activated by emotional situations or events), tends to be both smaller (13 percent smaller) and more reactive among people with BPD (Ruocco, Amirthavasagam, and Zakzanis 2012). This means that your amygdala may be similar to a small but very powerful sports car engine, revving up very high when someone steps on the gas.

Another area of the brain related to BPD is the hypothalamic-pituitary-adrenal axis (HPA axis), which functions as your natural stress-response system, preparing your body to face stress. Some studies have also found (perhaps not surprisingly) that people with BPD have more activity in their HPA axis than people without BPD (Zimmerman and Choi-Kain 2009). Therefore, your body is much more likely to go into fight-or-flight mode even when you aren't facing a serious threat.

Finally, studies have also shown that people with BPD may have less activity in the prefrontal cortex when they face emotional situations (Ruocco, Amirthavasagam, Choi-Kain, et al. 2012). This is important, because if the amygdala is like a powerful car engine, the prefrontal cortex is like the brakes, slowing down the car and calming the activity of the amygdala. If your brakes don't function well, your car won't slow down when you need it to. Indeed, you might have experienced this with your emotions from time to time.

Childhood Maltreatment

When it comes to environmental factors in the development of BPD, scientists have zeroed in on childhood maltreatment as a key influence. Childhood maltreatment can take many forms, including being neglected, not receiving enough support, or being physically, emotionally, or sexually abused. As it turns out, many people with BPD have had a history of childhood neglect or abuse of some sort. In fact, over half of people with BPD have experienced some kind of childhood sexual abuse, often of a frequent nature (Zanarini et al. 2002). Adverse and traumatic experiences like childhood sexual abuse can make it difficult to trust and feel secure in relationships with other people and can also result in a lot of shame and negative thoughts about yourself. Even among people with BPD who haven't experienced outright abuse, many have experienced serious emotional or physical neglect. As a result, sometimes they didn't get the help or support they needed to develop healthy coping strategies, or they might have gotten the message that they weren't important or good enough to take care of. This can lead to difficulty in learning how to take care of yourself and even to self-hate.

Invalidating Environments

Another childhood factor that might contribute to BPD is invalidation (Linehan 1993a). An *invalidating environment* is one in which people dismiss, disregard, or criticize you for having the emotions you have. We've worked with many people with BPD who weren't allowed to express sadness or fear because this was considered a sign of weakness. We've worked with others who say that their parents didn't seem to know how to soothe or care for them when they were upset, or whose parents lost control in these situations. Invalidation also can involve people saying that your problems aren't as big or as important as you think they are. It's a lot like being inside a burning building and yelling for help, while the fireman outside says, "What are you so upset about? Just climb over the rubble and come on out!"

Another way the environment can be invalidating is if children receive support and attention only once in a while or when they're particularly upset. If you have to really lose it to get people to pay attention to you and give you the support and help you need, or if you never know whether or when you'll get the support you need, you might learn to express yourself in a really intense way, and that could extend to other relationships in adulthood. Alternatively, you might develop a tendency to desperately hold on to any support or help you can get.

Sometimes invalidation is more subtle. Marsha Linehan (1993a), developer of an effective therapy for BPD, has described individuals with BPD as being like a rose in a tulip garden. In other words, people with BPD just feel different from other family members, being more emotional, intense, excitable, and so on. Your family may have been very well-intentioned and caring, but being surrounded by people who seem less emotional than you can make you feel as though there's something wrong with you or your emotions. For example, when a very emotional child wants something (such as a book or an activity, like going to the park), that desire can be so strong that it's almost like the child hasn't eaten for days and is seeing a plate of food held out of reach. If the child becomes extremely upset, others might be confused and inadvertently invalidate her or his pain because they have no idea what's going on or can't relate to the intensity of the child's feelings. We've spoken to many clients and families who have had such experiences.

The overall result of any form of abuse, neglect, or invalidation can be difficulties navigating close relationships and developing emotional bonds with others. You might feel very conflicted in relationships, desiring closeness but at the same time being terrified of intimacy or of losing the support of others. Both relationships and emotions might become very scary and seem fraught with danger. As mentioned, however, it probably takes more than just having an emotional temperament or growing up in a difficult, invalidating, or abusive environment for BPD to develop. We believe you need to have at least a couple of these factors, and that they all work together, much as a recipe will only yield certain results if specific ingredients (flour, baking soda, and so on) are combined in particular ways.

Different Pathways to BPD

In addition to the influences of brain, body, and environment and their interactions, there may be different pathways to developing BPD. Some people we've worked with have been through such horrendous stress, abuse, and invalidation that it seems nobody could have survived that environment without developing BPD. Others remember their childhood fondly and don't recall any trauma or abuse but do recall that they always felt very emotional, reactive, prone to stress, and different from other people.

We sometimes work with and educate family members, and we've heard the same types of things from them. Some family members we've worked with have been perplexed about the person's problems, saying that everything just changed dramatically for no apparent reason when the person entered early adolescence. Others have expressed strong guilt and remorse for the ways they or others treated the person as a child, and they struggle to come to terms with their role in the person's difficulties. To give you an idea of the diversity of potential pathways, the following sections provide a few examples of different ways in which people can develop BPD.

SAM

Sam grew up with two older sisters and one younger brother. Although life was chaotic in their household with four children, Sam remembers his childhood quite fondly and recalls that his parents and siblings were very kind and supportive. However, he felt like the black sheep in the family. He felt as if he was always the one who got upset, felt anxious about going to school, and was nervous around new people. He was also highly sensitive—not only to what people did or said, but to physical discomfort, such as tags on shirts and particular types of noises. Although Sam was an enthusiastic and boisterous child, his idiosyncrasies sometimes got on people's nerves, and his parents recalled days when he was a preschooler and threw one tantrum after another for hours on end.

Although Sam's family didn't seem to blame him for being so emotional, he did get the sense that he was the odd one out and that people were often fed up with him. He went through periods of overwhelming sadness and fear and didn't have any idea why. As he got older he had a few close friends, but he began to gravitate toward a group of kids who used drugs. He found that the thrill of his friendships with those risk takers, along with the highs of the drugs, temporarily drowned out his overwhelming emotions. Over time, he became hooked on increasingly dangerous drugs. He also began cutting himself after a particularly devastating breakup with a girlfriend when he was sixteen. At age twenty, he had been hospitalized twice for depression and suicide attempts, and a psychiatrist who met with him during one of his hospitalizations suggested that he might have BPD.

REBECCA

Rebecca grew up as an emotional child in a very difficult and stressful environment. Her parents had drug and alcohol problems, and she suffered severe neglect and emotional and physical abuse throughout her childhood. Although she was a bright and inquisitive child, she was hyperactive and had a difficult time focusing in the classroom, so she often felt inadequate

in comparison to her peers. She was diagnosed with a
deficit/hyperactivity disorder when she was in elementar
and needed extra help to get through the school day.

Rebecca remembered being a very intense and d
child, throwing frequent tantrums, and experiencing over
ing emotions, especially in close relationships. After her
passed away, she often took care of her father when he was
or hungover. In her teens, she frequently skipped school and
a variety of drugs, and she dropped out of school when sh
sixteen. Through her late teens, she attempted suicide se
times and burned and cut herself periodically. Although
stopped attempting suicide and found a job after she had her
son, she continued to drink heavily and often felt guilty
ashamed of herself as a parent. Finally, she began receiving l
from a mental health team and was diagnosed with BPD, alco
dependence, and post-traumatic stress disorder.

JAMIE

Jamie grew up in a family that "didn't do emotions." Althoug
he didn't remember himself being a particularly emotional child
and his uncles and cousins told him he had been pretty easygoing,
his parents had a hard time tolerating any expression of emotions.
He remembered that when he was a young boy, his father threw
him into a lake to retrieve something that had fallen off their
boat. Although he'd never had swimming lessons and didn't even
know how to tread water, his father left him in the water and kept
driving the boat forward. Jamie described this event as a meta-
phor for his whole childhood.

Jamie's parents were very strict and doled out physical punishment if Jamie didn't get straight As on his report card, got home later than his curfew, or supposedly talked back. As a result, he began to expect a lot of himself and often thought that if he didn't do something perfectly, he was a failure, despite being an extremely bright and capable student and an excellent athlete. He also suppressed his emotions much of the time, to the point where he felt as if he might explode. This made it hard for him to open up to others and express his thoughts, feelings, and opinions, and his relationships suffered as a result. Because he was so successful and hid his emotions so well, people didn't see the churning undercurrents below the seemingly calm surface he maintained. As a result, he rarely received the social and emotional support he needed from others, and he never learned to ask for it because doing so would be a shameful admission of his own inadequacy. When he snapped in his early twenties and was hospitalized for severe depression and suicidal thoughts, everyone was shocked.

MOVING FORWARD

Now that you know a little more about BPD and some of its possible causes, we hope that you feel empowered to take charge of your mental health and your recovery. The saying "Knowledge is power" is definitely true in regard to BPD, and the knowledge you've gained in your reading up to this point is the first step on your road to recovery. In chapter 3, we'll expand your knowledge even more by dispelling some of the common myths about BPD.

CHAPTER 3

BPD, MYTHS, AND
STIGMA: LEARNING THE
FACTS ABOUT BPD

When it comes to recovering from BPD, don't underestimate the power of knowing the facts. In the previous chapter, you learned about what BPD is and how it develops. However, another important step in learning about BPD is to debunk the myths that surround this disorder. Unfortunately, despite everything that has been learned about BPD since the 1990s, myths about this disorder persist. These myths muddy the waters of recovery, making it difficult to know the facts about BPD and get a clear sense of what you are facing. They also contribute to the fear and shame that some people experience when they are diagnosed with BPD.

So, what can you do to combat these myths? Well, as we mentioned in chapter 2, the saying "Knowledge is power" is key. The best way to fight misconceptions about BPD is to learn the facts about this disorder. Doing so can be an excellent first step in overcoming some of the shame, fear, or sadness you may be experiencing as a result of receiving this diagnosis.

In this chapter, we'll review some of the most common myths about BPD and provide you with the facts you need to combat these misconceptions. First, though, we want to discuss one of the main consequences of these misconceptions: stigma.

STIGMA

Stigma means associating negative qualities with someone simply because that person has a particular characteristic or condition, such as BPD. Stigma works a lot like stereotypes or racial prejudices, in that people start to judge everyone with a particular characteristic in the same unfavorable way. Stigma results in negative perceptions of any person who has that particular characteristic. When it comes to BPD, stigmatizing labels that have been attached to this disorder include "crazy," "violent," and "damaged," among others. You may have heard some of these judgments yourself. The problem is that these kinds of judgments are just assumptions that have nothing to do with the facts or the individual. Instead, they simply perpetuate misconceptions about BPD.

Stigma is a serious problem, and it has serious consequences. The stigma associated with BPD may prevent people from seeking the help they need or cause them to leave treatment prematurely (Sirey et al. 2001). Stigma can also influence how people think and feel about themselves (Link et al. 2001; Markowitz 1998). In fact, some of the biggest problems arise when stigma is internalized and people start to believe the negative judgments. Think about it: Even when you have the facts about BPD, recovering from this disorder is still a challenging process. BPD and the problems that often go along with this disorder are enough to deal with on their own. You don't need more problems added to your plate, particularly when those additional problems are negative judgments that equate you and your worth as a person with some of the symptoms you are struggling with.

There's a big difference between thinking, *When I'm angry, I sometimes do things that I later regret and don't understand* as opposed to *I'm crazy and out of control.* When you start to buy into negative judgments about BPD, it can lead to feelings of shame and self-blame. You may start to believe that your problems are your fault or that you don't deserve to get better. You may even question whether recovery is possible. If you've had any of these thoughts, or if you've judged yourself for having BPD, then you probably know how devastating this can be and how it can make recovery even more challenging. Therefore, getting the facts you need to combat these judgments is particularly important.

So, where does this stigma come from? There are several sources. The first has to do with the fact that BPD hasn't always been well understood, and unfortunately, people often respond most negatively to things they don't understand. In addition, many of the behaviors that go along with BPD can be shocking and confusing to others. Self-harm and suicide attempts, for example, may scare or confuse people. It's often difficult for someone who hasn't engaged in these behaviors to understand why people would hurt themselves. When people don't understand a behavior, and especially when that behavior scares them, it's often easier to judge the person who is engaging in that behavior than it is to make an effort to understand what's going on.

Another source of stigma is that some of the symptoms of BPD seem to conflict with characteristics viewed as optimal in our society. For example, our culture tends to value being "calm, cool, and collected" and "in control"—characteristics that stand in stark opposition to the intense emotions and difficulties regulating emotions that often accompany BPD.

Finally, a major source of stigma is the media, such as television and film. Because the media is so pervasive in our society, its impact is particularly powerful and far-reaching. And, for better or worse, the media seems drawn to BPD. Now, media attention in and of itself isn't necessarily a problem. Some shows have depicted problems such as self-harm in ways that promote understanding of this behavior and decrease the stigma associated with it. However, many films and television shows depict BPD in a sensationalized, overly simplistic, and negative manner. Let's face it: the media isn't known for its accurate and sensitive portrayal of complex problems, and BPD is no exception. The problem is that these negative portrayals reinforce stereotypes about BPD and perpetuate the misconceptions that so many researchers, clinicians, and advocacy groups are working hard to correct.

COMMON MYTHS ABOUT BPD

Although the stigma that surrounds BPD is a serious problem, it's a problem that can be solved. And the good news is that the best solution is a simple one: get the facts! To assist you with this, the following sections discuss some of the most common and pervasive myths about BPD, as well as the facts you need to combat them.

Myth 1: People with BPD Are Manipulative and Attention Seeking

The idea that people with BPD are manipulative and attention seeking may be one of the most common myths associated with BPD. Although it's not entirely clear where this myth came from, it probably grew out of a misguided attempt to explain some of the behaviors associated with BPD that can be difficult to comprehend, such as self-harm and suicide attempts. As we mentioned previously, for people who haven't struggled with these types of behaviors personally, they can be very shocking and lead to a variety of intense emotional responses, such as fear, anger, guilt, or confusion. In addition, because these behaviors are so serious and life threatening, many people want to intervene quickly to help or support the person who engages in them.

Although it may seem strange, it is this very desire to help that may have led to the myth that people with BPD are manipulative. Think about it this way: If you found yourself jumping to attention and helping someone under such dire circumstances (which is perfectly natural), you might erroneously conclude that the person became suicidal or engaged in self-harm on purpose to get your help or attention. As a result, you might feel as if you were "manipulated" into helping.

The problem is, just because a behavior has a particular outcome doesn't mean that the person engaging in that behavior planned it out and did it on purpose for that reason. Here's an example: Let's say you're playing a game of catch with some friends. Someone throws you the ball and you toss it to someone else. However, that person isn't paying attention and gets knocked in the head by the ball. Based on this outcome, we could say that you threw the ball with the intention of hitting that person in the head. Obviously, that would be a ridiculous conclusion. You can't infer a person's intentions based on the outcome or effect of her or his behavior.

The same principle applies to BPD. Although self-harm or suicide attempts may get people's attention or cause others to provide help, that doesn't mean that this is why the person engaged in these behaviors to begin with. There are many reasons people hurt themselves that have nothing to do with receiving attention or support. In fact, many people who engage in self-harm go to great lengths to try to hide this behavior from others—something that clearly contradicts this myth. Moreover, the most common reason people report for attempting suicide or harming themselves is to escape unbearable emotional pain, not to get support or attention from others.

What's more, even if people have learned that the only way to get attention from others is to engage in a behavior as extreme as self-harm, the fact that they resort to this behavior doesn't mean that they are manipulative. It may simply mean that they're desperately in need of some kind of attention, positive or negative, from another human being and don't know any other way to get that need met. The need for attention and support is common to all human beings, and not having this need met can be extremely painful. Assigning the label "manipulative" to someone who engages in self-harm or suicidal behaviors in an attempt to get needed care or attention ignores the fact that this is a basic human need.

Myth 2: People with BPD Are Violent and Dangerous

Another common myth is that people with BPD are violent. To put it simply, this myth is just plain wrong. Despite the tendency of some television series and films to portray people with BPD as violent criminals, the truth is that most people with BPD are actually at low risk for hurting others. Look at it this way: Violent behavior puts relationships in jeopardy and runs counter to the strong desire of people with BPD to be loved and accepted. It is also generally incompatible with the high sensitivity to the feelings of others that often goes along with BPD. Finally, given that one of the symptoms of BPD is a fear of abandonment, many people with BPD go to great lengths to preserve their relationships, even if it means sacrificing their own needs and desires in order to please others.

Now, this doesn't mean that people with BPD don't experience anger, or that they always express their anger effectively.

Because people with BPD tend to experience their emotions intensely, the anger they experience can be very strong and there may be times when they do or say things they later regret. However, research generally shows that people with BPD are more likely to take their anger out on themselves than on others. In fact, one of the reasons people with BPD engage in self-destructive behaviors is to punish themselves, which is a lot like taking anger out on themselves (Brown, Comtois, and Linehan 2002). The tendency to direct anger inward, rather than outward toward others, is one of the primary factors that distinguishes BPD from another personality disorder: antisocial personality disorder.

It's also important to remember that many people with BPD are actually "anger-phobic," or scared of the experience and expression of anger. This is most common among those who have witnessed or experienced firsthand extensive physical abuse and violence. Because behaviors such as these often occur in the context of anger, anger and violence may seem to go hand in hand for people who have had these types of experiences. As a result, they may end up being afraid of anger and avoiding it at all costs, partly to avoid inflicting such harm on others.

Myth 3: BPD Is Untreatable and a Life-Sentence

Because BPD is a personality disorder, many people (including some clinicians) mistakenly believe that the symptoms of BPD are part and parcel of who someone is. Therefore, one misconception is that anyone diagnosed with BPD will struggle with these symptoms forever. This is also one reason some clinicians used to believe that BPD couldn't be treated. Viewing the symptoms of BPD as a stable characteristic, much like someone's gender or ethnic background, didn't leave a lot of hope that these symptoms could be changed or alleviated. The good news is that this couldn't be further from the truth.

Research indicates that BPD actually has a very good prognosis—far better than was once believed. One of the most well-known studies in this area, and one of the largest studies to examine the course of BPD to date, has been following 290 patients with BPD (Zanarini et al. 2010). So far, over the first ten years of the study, 93 percent of the patients have gone at least two years without meeting criteria for BPD, and 86 percent have gone at least four years without meeting criteria for this disorder (Zanarini et al. 2010). The take-home message from this study is that BPD is not a chronic illness you have to live with for the rest of your life. Even though BPD is considered a personality disorder, this study shows that it is not a personality trait that never changes. Most people with BPD will go for years without struggling with these symptoms, and many will eventually make a full recovery.

In addition, a large body of research now shows that BPD is highly treatable and that there is great cause for hope. As it turns out, the belief that BPD couldn't be treated had more to do with the treatments being provided than the disorder itself. To put it quite simply, early treatments for BPD just weren't effective (Lieb et al. 2004). They weren't specialized to meet the needs of people with BPD or based on a good understanding of how BPD develops. Therefore, they just didn't work very well. Fortunately, there are now several effective treatments available for BPD, and a lot of evidence to suggest that people can make substantial progress in relatively short periods of time when treated with therapies developed specifically for this disorder (Bateman and Fonagy 1999; Gratz and Gunderson 2006; Linehan 1993a). Several treatments shown to be beneficial for people struggling with BPD are reviewed in chapter 4.

Myth 4: BPD Is Caused by Bad Parents

There was a time when "bad parenting" was thought to be the cause of many mental health problems. Although times have changed and most people now realize that the causes of any psychological disorder are far more complex, the myth that all people with BPD had bad, abusive, or neglectful parents persists.

In considering this myth, it's important to make a distinction between something that increases the chances of developing a disorder (a risk factor) and something that's necessary for the disorder to develop. When it comes to BPD, research has shown that negative childhood experiences, including childhood abuse and neglect, increase the risk for BPD (Zanarini 2000). However, not everyone with BPD has experienced childhood abuse or neglect, and not everyone who experiences childhood abuse or neglect develops BPD. Thus, although having a negative relationship with one's caregivers might increase the risk for BPD, it isn't necessary for the development of BPD and it definitely is not the sole cause of BPD. As we discussed in chapter 2, many other factors can contribute to the development of this disorder.

Indeed, the current understanding is that BPD probably arises from a combination of personality traits and stressful experiences during childhood. We use the broad term "stressful experiences" because research hasn't identified one specific type of stressful childhood experience that leads directly to the development of BPD. Therefore, even though these experiences can take the form of physical or sexual abuse or severe neglect, they can also take other forms, such as having a poor fit with your family or having caregivers who were often unavailable.

For example, if you have intense emotions (as most people with BPD do), then growing up in a family of people who don't experience their emotions intensely and are more even-keeled and low-key might have felt like a poor fit. You might have felt isolated, misunderstood, and as if you couldn't relate to anyone else in your family. If that was the case, then even if no one in your family ever told you that there was something wrong with having strong emotions, you might have felt like there was something wrong with you. Although this probably doesn't sound as severe as something like childhood abuse, feeling as if you're different from everyone else around you can be extremely stressful. And, in combination with certain personality traits and other stressful experiences, it could contribute to the development of BPD.

As another example, let's say you had caregivers who weren't always available—not because they were neglectful, but because they were busy with work or trying to make ends meet. Even though most of us would not label this "bad," as caregivers like these are clearly doing the best they can and probably have their children's best interests at heart, this could still be a stressful experience and leave a child with some unmet emotional needs.

The bottom line is that even though experiences of abuse, neglect, or invalidation may contribute to the development of BPD, they are in no way necessary for BPD to develop and also don't inevitably lead to BPD. In fact, in many cases, family members of people with BPD work incredibly hard to help their loved one in any way they can.

Myth 5: People with BPD Are Crazy and Irrational

The idea that people with BPD are crazy and irrational is another myth that is often reinforced by media depictions of this disorder. However, we can assure you that this myth is completely wrong. Although some of the behaviors common in BPD may appear incomprehensible to people who have never struggled with the intense emotions that go along with BPD, all of these behaviors serve a purpose in the moment and all are done to meet basic human needs. Ultimately, everything humans do serves some kind of purpose (whether we're aware of that purpose or not), and people with BPD are no exception to this rule. The only difference is that the types of behaviors necessary to obtain relief from very intense emotions are typically more extreme than those needed to relieve less intense emotions. Let's face it: You need a much warmer, tougher winter coat in the Arctic than you do in Hawaii. Therefore, although it may seem like some of the behaviors that go along with BPD, such as self-harm, drug use, or binge eating, don't make much sense, we can assure you that they actually serve an important purpose in the moment.

Likewise, although some of the thoughts that people with BPD experience may seem irrational to others, they are actually quite understandable and reasonable. Just like emotions and behaviors, thoughts don't pop up randomly out of the blue; they occur for a reason and make sense when you consider where they come from. For example, people with BPD often fear being abandoned or rejected by others. They may also worry that others will harm them in some way. Although these thoughts may not always be accurate in the present moment, chances are they are based on past experiences and were accurate in the past. The thoughts we have and the ways in which we evaluate situations, others' behaviors, and ourselves all have their origins in our life experiences.

Many people with BPD have experienced rejection or abandonment, sometimes when they most needed help or support. As a result, it's only natural that they might expect (or fear) this treatment from others. Viewing these thoughts as irrational dismisses their basis in real-world events and denies the painful experiences that many people who struggle with BPD have lived through.

The bottom line is that people with BPD are not inherently different from other people. The personality traits associated with BPD are the same traits that other people have; they may just be more pronounced or elevated in those with BPD. Likewise, the emotions experienced by people with BPD are the same emotions experienced by all human beings; they're just likely to be more intense and frequent in BPD. In the end, though, these are basic human experiences, with the primary difference being that the volume is turned up in BPD.

Myth 6: BPD Occurs Only in Women

There was a time when BPD was rarely diagnosed in men, and the common belief was that few men struggled with this disorder. This led to the myth that BPD is a disorder that afflicts only women. As more research was conducted, however, it became clear that men can and do develop BPD, and that the symptoms of this disorder are similar across genders. Yet, even with increasing awareness that BPD can occur in men, there was still a lot of evidence that BPD was diagnosed more often in women (Gunderson 2001). Therefore, many people continued to assume that BPD was much more common in women than in men. Thanks to continuing research in this area, however, we now have evidence that even this assumption may have been wrong. Specifically, a large study published in 2008 found that BPD occurs at similar rates among men and women (Grant et al. 2008). Thus, the take-home message regarding this myth is that BPD is an equal opportunity disorder that doesn't discriminate on the basis of gender.

MOVING FORWARD

We hope that this chapter has helped debunk some of the common myths about BPD and reduce the stigma associated with having a BPD diagnosis. Obviously, this was not a complete list of myths about BPD, and there are probably many others that we didn't address. If you encounter other myths about BPD that we didn't discuss here, we encourage you to address them head on by seeking accurate information. Research on BPD is growing at a rapid pace and doing wonders to increase people's knowledge about BPD. And, in the end, it is knowledge that will ultimately conquer misconceptions about BPD.

As you move forward in your recovery, keep in mind the facts we reviewed in this chapter. Perhaps most importantly, remember that BPD is a very human disorder. The symptoms of BPD don't stem from maliciousness, irrationality, or disregard for others; rather, they arise largely from understandable (albeit sometimes misguided) attempts to meet basic human needs. Take steps to learn as much as you can about BPD, and share the knowledge you gain with others. The more people know about BPD, the sooner we can get rid of the stigma associated with this disorder.

CHAPTER 4

EFFECTIVE TREATMENTS FOR BPD

Now that you know some of the key facts about BPD, we hope you can see that there are many reasons to be hopeful about this diagnosis. In this chapter, we discuss one of the most compelling reasons to be optimistic: treatments for BPD work! Despite past misconceptions that BPD is difficult or impossible to treat, a large body of recent scientific evidence indicates that treatment for BPD can be highly effective. In this chapter, we'll discuss the types of treatments available and their effectiveness. We'll also provide practical advice on getting the help you need.

IMPORTANT POINTS ABOUT TREATMENT

Before we delve into the details about treatments for BPD, here are some highlights for quick reference:

- Several psychological treatments for BPD have been proven highly effective. We'll briefly describe these treatments in this chapter so you'll know a bit about what to expect in each.

- Experts recommend that therapy for BPD be structured, organized, and aimed at helping you reduce self-destructive behaviors and improve your understanding and regulation of emotions and your ability to navigate relationships with others. The therapeutic relationship should be strong, compassionate, and validating.

- Because BPD is a complex disorder, the course of treatment is often longer (typically six months or more) than treatments for other problems, such as anxiety disorders or depression. However, people often experience significant reductions in symptoms within the first four to six months.

- The medications for BPD with the strongest scientific support include certain mood-stabilizing and antipsychotic medications.

- Medications are not necessary for recovery from BPD but can be helpful for some people. If you opt to take medication for BPD, it's best to receive some sort of therapy as well.

PSYCHOLOGICAL TREATMENTS AND THERAPY

Below, we describe some of the psychological treatments for BPD that have the most scientific evidence for their effectiveness. Keep in mind that the field is always moving forward, with old treatments becoming better and new treatments springing up, so this is just a snapshot of where things stand right now.

Dialectical Behavior Therapy

Developed by Marsha Linehan at the University of Washington, dialectical behavior therapy (DBT) is based on what is called the biosocial theory of BPD. In line with our discussion of causes of BPD in chapter 2, this theory posits that people with BPD have highly emotional temperaments and were raised in invalidating environments that didn't help them learn how to deal with their strong emotions. As a result, people with BPD often find their emotions to be confusing, overwhelming, and intolerable and may not trust how they feel. Therefore, one of the primary goals of DBT is to help people learn how to better understand, accept, and manage their emotions; this is called *emotion regulation*. DBT is made up of several different components:

- Weekly individual therapy focused on helping people change long-standing patterns of behavior, reduce self-destructive behaviors, and work toward important life goals

- Availability of an individual therapist for between-session coaching by phone, e-mail, or text-messaging, (the type of communication will depend on therapist and client preferences) to help people apply the new coping skills and strategies learned in therapy to everyday life·

- A weekly skills training group where people learn new ways to understand and manage emotions (emotion regulation skills), how to pay attention to the here and now (mindfulness skills), how to get through crises and overwhelming situations without making things worse (distress tolerance skills), and how to effectively navigate interactions with other people and use assertiveness to get needs met (interpersonal effectiveness skills)

- Weekly meetings of DBT therapists to help them continue to provide effective treatment and maintain their motivation and compassion

DBT is a form of cognitive behavioral therapy and involves lots of homework assignments, learning new skills, and working to change your behaviors. You might think of it as more of a "doing" or action-oriented approach to therapy.

Among the psychological and medical treatments for BPD, dialectical behavior therapy currently has the most scientific evidence. As of the writing of this book, fifteen rigorous scientific studies (randomized controlled trials) have tested the effectiveness of DBT for borderline personality disorder and various related problems (see Stoffers et al. 2010). From these studies, we know that DBT is especially effective at reducing suicidal and self-harming behavior, substance use problems, hospitalization and emergency room visits, and depression, and at increasing clients' functioning in daily life. Other research (Lynch et al. 2007; Robins and Chapman 2004) has shown that DBT can be effective for binge eating disorder and bulimia and the treatment of depression among older adults, and that the effects of DBT persist in the years following treatment. Anecdotally, many clients have told us that DBT has been a very important part of their journey to recovery.

Mentalization-Based Treatment

Like DBT, mentalization-based treatment (MBT) involves weekly individual and group therapy sessions. MBT is based on the theory that we all need consistent input from our caregivers in order to learn about our own and others' thoughts and feelings and develop a consistent sense of who we are. This works best when our parents or caregivers express interest in how and why we feel the way we do and mirror our emotions back to us. For example, if a child is with his mother and begins to cry, she might say, "Oh, are you sad? What happened? Why are you sad?" In this interaction, the child's sadness is reflected back, or mirrored, by his mother, and he learns that crying might indicate sadness.

These types of experiences help children develop the ability to mentalize, or understand that their own behaviors and the behaviors of others arise from internal, mental states, such as thoughts, feelings, and desires. If you have BPD, you may have missed out on these types of interactions, and as a result, your actions and those of other people may seem to come from out of the blue. You may also be confused about your thoughts and feelings and who you really are as a person—your sense of self. MBT therapists use two primary approaches to help people develop the ability to mentalize:

- Weekly individual therapy sessions focused on helping people understand why they do what they do, what might drive the actions of other people, and the links between thoughts, feelings, and behaviors

- Weekly group therapy focused on helping all members of the group consider their own and others' mental states and how these relate to behaviors. Group members and leaders try their best to understand how their behaviors affect the mental states (thoughts, feelings, and desires) and behaviors of other group members, and vice versa.

One of the things that makes MBT very different from DBT is that MBT is a psychoanalytic treatment, not a cognitive behavioral treatment. In other words, MBT is more of a talk therapy than DBT. If you engage in MBT, most of your time will be spent talking with your therapist and learning about yourself and your relationships with other people. Although you might walk away from MBT with some of the same skills taught in DBT, you would learn them in a very different way.

In two large studies (Bateman and Fonagy 1999, 2008, 2009) of two different forms of MBT—an outpatient treatment and an eighteen-month form that includes partial hospitalization—this approach has shown promise in reducing suicide attempts, self-harm, depression, and anxiety and in improving relationships and general social functioning. Moreover, one of these studies indicated that MBT has some excellent long-term effects, with many of the treatment gains being maintained over a five-year follow-up period after treatment (Bateman and Fonagy 2008).

Other Psychological Treatments

In addition to DBT and MBT, other psychological treatments can help you along the path to recovery. We focused on DBT and MBT because the evidence for these treatments is the strongest. Other treatments that have been proven helpful for people with BPD are schema-focused therapy, transference-focused psychotherapy, and emotion regulation group therapy (Gratz and Gunderson 2006; Gratz and Tull 2011).

- In schema-focused therapy, you meet three times a week with a therapist for individual treatment focused on helping you understand your typical thought patterns, such as thoughts of worthlessness, rejection, or self-hatred. You'll also look at how you learned these ways of thinking and learn how to free yourself from them.

- Transference-focused psychotherapy is a psychodynamic treatment, meaning that it focuses on your ongoing relationship with your therapist, your emotional reactions and thoughts in therapy sessions, and your past experiences with people close to you, such as your parents or siblings.

- Emotion regulation group therapy is a fourteen-week group treatment designed to reduce self-harm and other self-destructive behaviors by teaching more adaptive ways of responding to and regulating your emotions.

The Good News and the Bad News about Psychological Treatments

The good news is that there are effective psychological treatments for BPD. The bad news is that these treatments may not be available in your community. Now for more good news: All of these treatments have important points in common, so if you can't find someone who practices a certain form of therapy, treatment can still be highly effective if it includes these common elements. If you're unable to find a therapist specializing in one of the treatments outlined above, look for one who can provide the common elements that most experts agree should be part of treatment for BPD:

- Treatment should be structured and organized. People with BPD (and many others) do much better with treatments and therapy sessions that are structured. In practical terms, this means therapy sessions shouldn't simply be open-ended discussions of your problems; rather, they should have a clear agenda or game plan and a start and stop time, and should address your difficulties in an organized, logical, and systematic way.

- Treatment should help you reduce impulsive or self-destructive behaviors, such as self-harm, suicide attempts, drug use, and so on. This may seem obvious, but continuing to engage in self-destructive behaviors can make it very difficult to recover.

- Treatment should also teach you strategies to manage your emotions more effectively and resolve any major life issues that are contributing to your difficulties. If you remain miserable, simply stopping self-harming behaviors won't suffice.

- Treatment should address interpersonal and relationship difficulties. Many people with BPD have significant relationship difficulties, and it's awfully hard to build a life that works well and is satisfying if your relationships are in turmoil. Indeed, for many people connections with others are one of the most important building blocks in a fulfilling and happy life.

- The therapist or treatment provider should be skilled at expressing empathy, validation, and compassion, and at developing a strong working therapeutic relationship. It's difficult to progress in therapy if you think your therapist doesn't understand or care about you. Conversely, a strong, positive therapeutic relationship can play an important and memorable role along your road to recovery.

MEDICATION

Psychotropic medications (basically, drugs with psychological, emotional, or behavioral effects) are often used to help people with BPD. Generally, medication treatments are based on the idea that you may have an imbalance in *neurotransmitters* (chemical messengers that make your brain work). For example, the category of medications known as selective serotonin reuptake inhibitors help keep levels of the neurotransmitter serotonin higher, enhancing mood and preventing or decreasing impulsive actions.

Several different types of medications are used to treat symptoms of BPD—primarily antidepressants, mood-stabilizing medications, and antipsychotics. Below, we discuss medications in each category and their effectiveness.

Antidepressants

Antidepressants work by increasing the availability of several different types of neurotransmitters in the brain, including serotonin, norepinephrine, and dopamine. Although there are many different types of antidepressants, research has failed to show consistent or strong evidence for positive effects of antidepressants for patients with BPD (Lieb et al. 2010). Among the most commonly used antidepressants are selective serotonin reuptake inhibitors (SSRIs), including citalopram (Celexa), escitalopram (Lexapro), fluoxetine (Prozac), fluvoxamine (Luvox), paroxetine (Paxil), and sertraline (Zoloft). A small amount of research has shown that SSRIs may be helpful in reducing depression, anxiety, and mood shifts among people with BPD (Lieb et al. 2010). SSRIs also tend to have the fewest serious side effects of the antidepressant medications, although it is important to know that not everyone can tolerate SSRIs.

Despite having the fewest serious side effects, SSRIs do come with long lists of more minor side effects that are fairly common, including nausea, diarrhea, headaches, anxiety, nervousness, sleep disturbance, restlessness and agitation, fatigue, dizziness, light-headedness, sexual problems (including lower sex drive), tremor, dry mouth, sweating, weight loss or gain, rashes, and seizures. It typically takes three to six weeks for antidepressants, including SSRIs, to have noticeable effects, so if you're trying out this type of medication, you may need to be patient; it could take a while to experience changes in your mood, energy level, or depression. Finally, for some people antidepressants may increase the risk of suicidal behavior. Although this is usually temporary, it's important to be alert to this possibility.

Mood-Stabilizing Medications

With mood instability being such an important and troublesome symptom of BPD, it makes a lot of sense that mood stabilizers are sometimes prescribed for people with BPD. These medications tend to work by changing brain chemistry in a way that evens out moods, both high and low. Examples of mood stabilizers include lithium, carbamazepine (Tegretol), gabapentin (Neurontin), lamotrigine (Lamictal), oxcarbazepine (Trileptal), topiramate (Topamax), and valproate or divalproex (Depakote). There is some evidence that certain mood stabilizers may be helpful in the treatment of some of the emotional and interpersonal symptoms that go along with BPD (Lieb et al. 2010).

Mood stabilizers may be most effective if you've been diagnosed with both BPD and *bipolar disorder*, a condition that involves extreme mood shifts from periods of depression to periods of mania or hypomania (a less intense form of mania). Lithium has some fairly common side effects, including nausea, hand tremors, increased urination, diarrhea, upset stomach, increased thirst, and decreased appetite. In addition, when taking lithium, you have to monitor your diet and ensure that you're on the correct dose, as high doses can be toxic. Divalproex shouldn't be taken if you're pregnant. It also has a number of troubling side effects, including irritability, hair loss, reduced platelet count (which leads to easy bruising), liver toxicity, and pancreatitis (inflammation of the pancreas).

Antipsychotic Medications

When you read the term "antipsychotic medications," you might think, *I'm not psychotic! What do you mean "antipsychotics"?* While antipsychotics are indeed used for people with schizophrenia, hallucinations, delusions, and other such symptoms, they are also helpful for a variety of other concerns, including BPD. Generally speaking, the newer antipsychotics work by reducing the availability of the neurotransmitter dopamine (which is involved in mood, pleasure, and body movement) in certain areas of the brain. There are several different types of antipsychotics, but the most common medications in the newer generation include aripiprazole (Abilify), clozapine (Clozaril), loxapine (Loxitane), olanzapine (Zyprexa), risperidone (Risperdal), and sertindole (Serlect). Studies have investigated the use of several different types of antipsychotics for BPD, and the most consistent evidence suggests that aripiprazole (Abilify) may help with several symptoms of BPD, including anger, impulsivity, and interpersonal problems. Although there has been some favorable evidence for olanzapine (Zyprexa), other evidence suggested that this medication may actually increase risk of self-harming behaviors (Lieb et al. 2010).

Some of the most common side effects of antipsychotics include sedation or fatigue, low blood pressure, weight gain, temperature increases or decreases (for example, feeling hot a lot of the time), changes in the activity of the heart and cardiovascular system, and changes in skin pigmentation. More serious side effects, which occur infrequently, include tardive dyskinesia (a disorder involving involuntary movements) and neuroleptic malignant syndrome (muscular rigidity, elevated temperature, blood pressure increases or decreases, and a sense of altered consciousness). If you are taking an antipsychotic and experience symptoms of either of these conditions, contact your doctor immediately.

LEVELS OF TREATMENT

Thus far, we've described outpatient treatments, but other levels of treatment are available. Outpatient treatment involves seeing a therapist or other mental health treatment provider while living at home, attending sessions in a medical or clinic setting, and possibly medications. It may also include case management, to help you deal with issues of daily living. More intensive treatments might include an extended stay at a psychiatric hospital, where you live at the hospital for a while and often receive a combination of both medication and psychological care. If your problems are on the more severe end of the spectrum, you might want to consider more intensive or more involved treatment. In this case, we strongly recommend that you talk with your psychiatrist or mental health professional about your options. But to give you an idea of what you might try, here are some possibilities.

If you have persistent difficulties with everyday living issues, such as housing, finances, employment, hygiene, severe isolation, or symptoms such as hallucinations or serious delusions, we recommend that you consider a combination of care that includes regular therapy, medication services, and possibly case management services to assist you with the daily living issues. It can be hard to benefit from therapy if some of the foundations of your life are unsteady, so you may need help in stabilizing your situation before you can really work on recovery from BPD.

If you also have bipolar disorder and you haven't done so already, we recommend that you visit a psychiatrist for a medication evaluation. Medication can be very effective in helping people with bipolar disorder even out their moods and in preventing some of the problems that arise during manic episodes, such as out-of-control behavior and overspending.

If you're having tremendous difficulty keeping yourself safe and not seriously harming yourself or others, it may be helpful to consider at least short-term inpatient care, partial hospitalization, or a day treatment program if these services are available in your community. These alternatives may also be helpful if you've tried therapy and just can't seem to get yourself to leave your home or participate in therapy sessions. That said, we've seen many people who struggle with these issues, having trouble stopping themselves from attempting suicide or having urges to harm others, who manage to do quite well and experience major improvements in outpatient treatment, sometimes in combination with medication.

Provided that you don't require a more intrusive type of treatment, we normally recommend that people start with the least intensive and life-altering options, such as regular outpatient therapy, psychiatric care, or both. We also recommend that if you're taking medication, you receive psychological treatment or therapy of some sort.

CASEY'S STORY

Casey had a history of serious alcohol problems, self-injury, and suicide attempts and also experienced intense social anxiety, avoiding people and groups much of the time but then becoming involved in risky sexual activity and dangerous encounters with men while she was drinking. After being diagnosed with BPD, she was unsure whether regular outpatient DBT would be enough for her, but she decided to give it a try. DBT involved attending individual treatment sessions and a therapy group designed to help her learn new coping skills. She attended two group sessions but experienced such intense panic attacks that she was reluctant to return.

In her individual treatment, the therapist helped her reduce self-harming behaviors, and Casey almost completely stopped drinking for several weeks. However, despite all her efforts, her problems with drinking soon returned, she began to make more suicide attempts, and her self-harming behaviors increased again. She also had difficulty leaving her home and maintaining her daily hygiene and self-care. As a result, she and her case manager decided that she needed an extra boost of treatment. She got a referral for a sixty-day inpatient treatment program. After this treatment, and after having been away from alcohol and not engaging in self-destructive behaviors, she was ready to return to therapy and group sessions. Although she still struggled with intense anxiety and fought urges to drink and engage in self-harming behaviors on a daily basis, she was able to jump into therapy with both feet the second time around and gradually noticed significant improvements in her life.

MOVING FORWARD

The bottom line is that treatment for BPD can be very effective, and several different types of treatments—both psychological and pharmaceutical—are backed up by solid scientific evidence. In terms of psychological treatments, DBT has the most evidence, but in recent years several other types of therapy have been developed and appear to be very promising. Keep in mind that therapy is more likely to work if you take an active role, asking your treatment provider for information, working together on therapy goals that are important to you, and incorporating what you learn in therapy into your daily life.

In terms of medications, those with the most solid evidence for treating BPD are certain mood stabilizers and antipsychotics. Most experts would recommend, however, that you avoid relying solely on medications. Always supplement medications with some form of therapy. One final suggestion is that you view treatment as a way to build the life you want. As is sometimes said in DBT, the goal of therapy is a life worth living (Linehan 1993a). Even when times are extremely difficult and your situation seems unbearable, keep reminding yourself to stay on the path toward a life worth living. Given how many effective treatments there are for BPD, we're confident that you'll have a lot of support and success on your road to recovery.

CHAPTER 5

※——※

FINDING TREATMENTS
FOR BPD

As we discussed in the previous chapter, there are many effective treatments for BPD, and many reasons to be hopeful about your ability to recover from this disorder. However, the fact that help exists doesn't mean it's always easy to find. For many people, finding help for BPD can be a daunting experience. You may not know where to turn or what options are available to you. You might even feel overwhelmed or paralyzed at the prospect of starting this process. If you've been unsure about how to find the help you need, consider this chapter your guide.

In this chapter, we'll give you tips on where to start and how to find the help you need, as well as some pointers on how to determine which treatment is best for you. We hope this alleviates some of the stress that often goes along with seeking treatment for BPD.

IDENTIFYING TREATMENT OPTIONS IN YOUR AREA

One of the biggest hurdles in finding treatment for BPD is figuring out which treatment options are available in your area. It can be frustrating to learn that there are effective treatments for BPD but not know whether they're available in your area or how to go about finding them. The good news is that there are resources that can help with this.

Start with the Person Who Made the Diagnosis

One good starting point is the person who diagnosed you with BPD. Ask this person for treatment recommendations, including where to seek treatment and the best options available in your area. More often than not, if a mental health professional has diagnosed you with BPD, that person will have a good understanding of the symptoms you're struggling with and the types of treatments you may need. Even if the person who diagnosed you doesn't specialize in the treatment of BPD, she or he will probably be able to recommend professionals who do, or who work with clients with the particular difficulties you are struggling with, such as self-harm or disordered eating behaviors. Even if it has been a while since you received your diagnosis, it's perfectly fine to contact the clinician who diagnosed you and ask for treatment referrals. That's part and parcel of conducting diagnostic assessments, so don't hesitate to reach out and ask for help.

Local Resources

If you didn't receive your BPD diagnosis from a mental health professional and have not yet met with a clinician to confirm this diagnosis, or if the clinician who diagnosed you with BPD isn't able to provide you with information on BPD treatment resources in your area, have no fear. There are other local resources you can contact to find treatment options in your area, including psychological associations, universities, mental health organizations, and treatment centers.

One useful source of information is your state or provincial psychological or psychiatric association. These associations can give you information on treatment providers in your area, and many provide referral services. Therefore, it's always a good idea to contact those organizations and inquire about professionals who specialize in the treatment of BPD.

If you live in the United States, you might also want to contact your state chapter of the National Alliance on Mental Illness (NAMI) to see whether they have any information on local BPD treatment providers or other ideas on how you can find the treatment you need. NAMI is an organization dedicated to helping consumers get the best treatment available for a range of mental health problems. Therefore, they are often familiar with local treatment options and also strongly committed to helping people get the care they need.

College and university psychology departments, counseling centers, and psychology training clinics can also be useful resources. Even if you don't receive services from the university clinic or counseling center, they will often have listings of appropriate referrals in your area.

Another option is to contact a mental health professional or intake coordinator within the Department of Psychiatry at your local hospital or medical center. These individuals usually have a fair amount of knowledge about local treatment resources and may be able to point you in the right direction. In many communities, clinicians, researchers, and faculty members working in mental health know each other or, at the very least, know of one another. Therefore, any of these people may be able to provide you with information on resources in your area.

Use the Internet—Selectively

Another source of information on BPD treatment providers is the Internet. As we discussed in chapter 1, although it's best to be cautious when using the Internet to find information on BPD, some websites are trustworthy, and these generally offer excellent resources for finding BPD treatment providers. For example, the website for Behavioral Tech, LLC, the company Dr. Marsha Linehan founded to train mental health professionals in DBT and other evidence-based treatments, has a directory of DBT therapists. (From the home page at www.behavioraltech.org, click on the "Find a DBT Therapist" link.) One thing to keep in mind if you use this directory is that it provides information only on clinicians who provide DBT. Therefore, there could be other treatment providers in your area who specialize in the treatment of BPD but are not listed in this directory.

Another helpful resource is the website for the Association for Behavioral and Cognitive Therapies (www.abct.org), which also provides a therapist directory. To access this directory, click on the "Find a Therapist" link on the web page. Although this directory doesn't allow you to search for treatment providers who specialize in BPD per se, it does allow you to search for treatment providers who have experience in DBT, as well as those who have experience treating behaviors common in BPD, such as self-injurious behaviors. As the name implies, the Association for Behavioral and Cognitive Therapies is made up of mental health professionals who have been trained in cognitive behavioral therapies. Therefore, if you are interested in finding someone who provides a treatment for BPD that isn't cognitive behavioral in nature, such as MBT or medication-focused treatment, this resource won't be as helpful.

A similar search engine is available at the website for the American Psychological Association (locator.apa.org). Although it also does not allow you to search for treatment providers who specialize in BPD, it does provide a list of treatment providers who specialize in the treatment of personality disorders in general. An added benefit of this search engine is that it also allows you to fine-tune your search by identifying psychologists who speak certain languages, are sensitive to specific cultural identities, or are of a particular gender or sexual orientation. Therefore, this search engine may help you find a therapist who is a good fit for you personally.

Finally, you may want to visit the website for the Treatment and Research Advancements National Association for Personality Disorder (www.tara4bpd.org). This organization was founded in 1994 by Valerie Porr and is dedicated to helping people with BPD and their loved ones obtain accurate information about this disorder. The website has excellent and up-to-date information on BPD and its treatment, and the organization also has a BPD hotline and referral center (1-888-482-7227). This is a great option if you don't have access to the Internet. The hotline is available Monday through Friday from 12 noon to 5 p.m. Eastern Standard Time and is an excellent source of information. The referral center can provide information on clinicians in your area who specialize in the treatment of BPD, as well as local support groups for yourself or your loved ones.

SELECTING A TREATMENT PROVIDER

Once you've identified BPD treatment providers in your area and have a sense of the treatment options available to you, it's important to figure out which type of mental health professional is likely to be the best fit for you. Several different types of mental health professionals may be qualified to treat BPD, including psychologists, psychiatrists, licensed mental health counselors, and licensed clinical social workers. In the following sections, we discuss how these different types of mental health providers differ from one another.

Psychologists

Psychologists are mental health professionals who have a PhD (doctor of philosophy) or PsyD (doctor of psychology) degree in either clinical or counseling psychology. In order to obtain one of these degrees, a person has to attend a graduate training program that generally lasts about five to six years and provides training in the assessment and psychological treatment of a variety of psychological disorders. Most graduate training programs also require a one-year, full-time internship that provides additional, hands-on experience in assessment and treatment.

Although psychologists receive a lot of training in the treatment of psychological disorders, graduate programs differ in the specific types of training they provide, and not all graduate programs or internships include training in the treatment of personality disorders. In addition, training programs differ in the types of treatments they emphasize, with some focusing primarily on cognitive behavioral treatments such as DBT, and others focusing more on psychodynamic or psychoanalytic approaches, such as MBT.

Psychiatrists

Psychiatrists are medical doctors with training in the treatment of psychiatric disorders. Just like psychologists, psychiatrists may receive training in a variety of different therapeutic approaches. Therefore, the type of treatment they provide will likely vary depending on the training they received, with some psychiatrists providing psychodynamic treatments and others offering cognitive behavioral treatments. In addition to receiving general medical training, the primary way that psychiatrists differ from psychologists is that they can prescribe psychiatric medications. If you are interested in medication treatments, you will probably need to work with a psychiatrist (although some psychologists in a few states in the United States are now allowed to prescribe medications as well).

Another thing to keep in mind is that psychiatrists vary in whether and to what extent they provide psychological treatments in addition to medication treatments. Some offer both psychological and medication treatments to their clients, so you could get all of the treatment you need from the same person. Others primarily offer medication treatments, so you would need to meet with someone else for psychological treatment. It's actually fairly common for people with BPD to work with both a psychiatrist and a psychologist or counselor.

Licensed Counselors and Social Workers

Finally, some mental health professionals have a master's degree in counseling psychology or social work. Most master's programs in these areas last about two years and provide training in the treatment of a variety of psychological disorders. Although not all social workers or counselors receive specialized training in working with certain disorders, such as BPD, some do, and others may obtain this training after receiving their degrees. People with a master's degree who are licensed to treat people will have a series of initials after their names, such as LCSW (licensed clinical social worker) or LMHC (licensed mental health counselor).

Choosing a Practitioner

So, which of these types of treatment providers is going to be the best fit for you? That depends on your needs and the type of treatment you're most interested in receiving. As we mentioned above, if you are interested in medication treatments, then you'll generally need to meet with a psychiatrist. If you're interested in psychological treatment, any of these types of treatment providers may be able to provide the treatment you want, depending on the specific types of training they've received.

One thing to keep in mind is that even though most mental health professionals will probably know what BPD is and the symptoms that go along with it, that doesn't mean they know how to treat BPD. Many mental health professionals don't receive specialized training in BPD and may not have much experience in working with clients with this disorder. Therefore, when selecting a treatment provider, it's a good idea to get information on the training and experience of all the mental health professionals you're considering.

Now, some people feel uncomfortable asking clinicians about their background and experience. We want to assure you that it's completely okay to do this. In fact, most clinicians expect it. Remember, you are a consumer seeking a service from a professional in your community. Just as you would want your mechanic to know how to fix a problem with your car's transmission, you would want a clinician to know how to diagnose and treat BPD. Therefore, you are completely within your rights to ask as many questions as you would like about someone's qualifications. You need to collect as much information as you can in order to make an informed choice. Here are some questions you may want to ask:

- Where did you receive your training?

- What kind of training have you had in the assessment and treatment of personality disorders?

- Did you receive specialize training in working with people who have BPD?

- Do you have training in DBT, MBT, or other empirically supported treatments for BPD?

- What kinds of treatment do you provide (for example, cognitive-behavioral, psychodynamic, DBT, or MBT)?

- How many years have you been working with clients in general and clients with BPD in particular?

- How many clients with BPD have you worked with?

- Are you licensed? If not, are you supervised by a licensed clinician?

- What is the cost of the treatment? Do you accept private insurance, Medicare, or Medicaid?

To download these questions in the form of a worksheet that you can print and take with you to consultations, please visit www.newharbinger.com/27060.

After you've identified a clinician who's qualified to treat BPD, the next step is to ask yourself whether you feel comfortable with this person. Treatment of BPD can be an intense and challenging process. For treatment to be most effective, it's important that you feel comfortable opening up and sharing painful thoughts, emotions, and experiences with your therapist. This doesn't necessarily have to happen right away; it's okay if it takes you a while to build a trusting relationship with your therapist. However, it's important that you feel safe with your therapist and believe that she or he has your best interests at heart even as you work toward building trust in this relationship.

Unfortunately, we can't offer any specific questions you can ask to determine whether you will feel comfortable with a given mental health professional. Sometimes even a well-qualified and highly trained therapist may not feel like a good fit for you. You might feel like you don't click with that person, or you might feel uncomfortable opening up to her or him. It really comes down to a gut feeling about how much you can trust the person. Sometimes the best source of information is your gut instinct, so trust your feelings.

It's also completely reasonable to look for a therapist with specific characteristics in addition to experience and training with BPD. For example, if you are a woman or if you have had negative experiences with men in the past, you may prefer to work with a female therapist. Making your preferences known when looking for a therapist and actively seeking a therapist of a particular gender is perfectly okay. As we mentioned above, it's important that you feel comfortable with your therapist, and, for many people, this means working with someone of a particular gender. You may also be interested in finding a therapist who shares other characteristics with you, like racial or ethnic background, sexual orientation, or religion. Once again, having these preferences and making them known is completely okay. In fact, it's so common that many therapists expect it.

That said, as much as we encourage you to share your preferences with potential treatment providers and to try to find the best fit for you, it may not be possible to find a therapist who is a perfect fit for you. Depending on where you live, you may not have a lot of options for BPD treatments. You may have to choose among just a few qualified professionals, or there may be only one professional qualified to treat BPD. The good news is that working with someone to whom you may not relate right away, or with whom you don't immediately feel comfortable, can be a great learning experience. It can teach you important skills in how to build relationships and provide opportunities to practice trusting others and tolerating uncertainty. Depending on your past experiences, it may also bring up painful emotions that are important to work through with your therapist in session. Doing this will strengthen your relationship with your therapist and enhance your progress in therapy.

In the end, our best advice is to keep an open mind when meeting with potential therapists and to be honest about any concerns you have about working with them. Expressing these concerns directly will provide you and your potential therapist with the opportunity to address these concerns directly and perhaps even alleviate them. Also, remember that therapists are usually accustomed to having these types of conversations with potential clients, and most therapists welcome the chance to improve the therapeutic relationship. So, consider this part and parcel of finding a treatment provider and speak up if you have any concerns.

FINDING MEDICATION TREATMENTS

When it comes to finding the right medication treatment, there are a few other things to keep in mind. The first question is whether you even want to take medications. As we discussed in chapter 4, several medications have been found to be helpful in addressing some of the symptoms of BPD, and many people with BPD are prescribed medications. However, that doesn't mean that medications are necessary for recovery from BPD. The most effective treatments for BPD are psychological treatments, so it's really up to you to determine whether you want to take medications. If you think you may want to give medication a try, we encourage you to discuss this with your treatment providers and explore your options. We also recommend that you take some time to identify the pros and cons of taking medications.

If you decide to pursue medication treatment, the first step is to meet with a psychiatrist or other medical professional for an assessment of your symptoms and medical history. This information will be used to select the medication that is likely to be best for you. Once you start taking the medication, it's important to meet with your prescribing physician regularly to monitor how well the medication is working and whether you are experiencing any side effects that may be cause for concern.

If you've already been to a psychiatrist, you may be familiar with psychotropic medications. Indeed, many people with BPD have been prescribed a number of different psychotropic medications even before they are diagnosed with BPD. Even if you've already been prescribed a psychotropic medication or have been taking medications for years, we still encourage you to have an open discussion with your treatment provider about the potential benefits and side effects of the medication you're taking.

We've provided some questions for you to ask your prescribing physician if you are currently taking medications, or if you are considering starting a new medication. They're also available online in the form of a printable questionnaire; please visit www.newharbinger.com/27060 to download it.

- What side effects are most common?

- Which side effects should I be concerned about if they occur?

- Did you consider other medications, and why did you choose this one for me?

- How well does this medication usually work for people with the types of difficulties I experience?

- Are there any medications, foods, drugs, or alcohol that I should avoid while taking this medication? Does this medication have any harmful interactions with any other medications or foods?

- When can I expect the medication to start working?

If you are currently taking psychotropic medications, or if you decide to begin medication treatment, it's important to follow your prescribing physician's orders with regard to when and how the medication should be taken. Some medications need to be taken in certain ways, or they can be ineffective or even harmful. By following your prescribing physician's orders, you'll give your medications the chance to work as well as they can.

TAKING AN ACTIVE ROLE IN YOUR TREATMENT

Once you begin working with a mental health professional, we recommend that you take an active role in your treatment. The first step is to seek information from your treatment provider so that you are completely clear about what to expect and what is required of you. Again, the best way to do this is to ask questions. Here are some examples of the types of questions you might ask:

- How well does this treatment work?

- How long do you expect treatment to last?

- What types of changes in my life can I expect?

- What is your policy about telephone calls, extra sessions, and emergencies?

- What can I do to make this treatment work best?

- What will I be asked to do outside of treatment?

- How often will we be meeting each week?

- How will sessions be structured?

- Are there any side effects of this treatment that I should look out for?

These questions are also available online in the form of a printable questionnaire. Visit www.newharbinger.com/27060 to download a copy.

Another way to take an active role in your treatment is to jump into it with both feet. As with many things in life, what you get out of treatment is going to be influenced by how much you put into it. And when it comes to treatment, this often involves doing things outside of the treatment sessions. A key part of many treatments for BPD is outside-of-session assignments, or homework. If you are new to treatment, you might be asking yourself, *Did I just read the word "homework"?* Indeed you did. Many treatments require you to do out-of-session assignments each week, and these treatments tend to be far more effective when people do their homework consistently and regularly practice the new skills they are learning.

Even if the treatment you choose doesn't involve homework, all treatments require you to make some changes in your life, whether in the way you act, think, deal with your emotions, interact with other people, or care for your body. Try your best to make these changes and follow your clinician's recommendations as closely as possible. Recovering from BPD requires that you take an active stance, so throw yourself into treatment and practice the new things you are learning, and we guarantee you will get the most out of your treatment.

MOVING FORWARD

Making the decision to get treatment for BPD and finding the right treatment for you is not an easy task. It can be very stressful, especially if you don't know where to start. Fortunately, there has been a lot of research conducted on this disorder and how best to treat it. As a result, mental health professionals now have a good sense of how to treat BPD. With each passing year, there are new developments in the treatment of BPD and more mental health professionals are receiving training in how best to treat individuals who struggle with this disorder. We hope this chapter can serve as your guide as you begin the process of finding the treatment that is best for you.

CHAPTER 6

※≫————————————————————————————※

HOW BPD AFFECTS
LOVED ONES AND HOW
TO GET THE SUPPORT
YOU NEED

Relationships with people who genuinely care for and support you can be crucial on your road to recovery from BPD, providing both the fuel to keep going and the shelter to help you weather storms along the way. Yet one of the major areas of difficulty in BPD involves instability in relationships. You might have noticed that sometimes holding on to the very things you need from those close to you, such as warmth, validation, caring, and support, is a lot like trying to hold sand in your hands: it keeps slipping through your fingers.

Making matters worse, some of the difficulties that come along with BPD, such as emotional ups and downs, intense anger, and suicidal and self-harming behavior, can be overwhelming and confusing for loved ones. And when people are overwhelmed and confused, they often aren't great at offering support. Maybe you've noticed that even those who are closest to you don't really get what you're going through, are stressed or burned-out, or say or do invalidating things on a regular basis. In this chapter, we'll discuss how difficulties related to BPD may be affecting loved ones and what you can do to interact with them more effectively. We hope it helps improve your relationships and allows you take the steps necessary to get the support you need.

COMMON EXPERIENCES OF LOVED ONES

We've done a fair amount of work with loved ones of those with BPD (and other mental health problems), and we've observed several common experiences and reactions. Generally speaking, fear, worry, and guilt are among the most common and upsetting experiences of loved ones, and we'll discuss those feelings in more detail below. More briefly, here are some of the other common reactions we've seen:

- Being confused about how your BPD developed or about when, how, or whether to talk with you about your difficulties

- Feeling helpless, powerless, and as though they can't do anything to help

- Feeling sadness and sorrow about the effects of BPD on your life

- Experiencing sadness and a feeling of loss regarding the life they had envisioned for you (particularly common for parents and caregivers)

- Feeling overwhelmed by the challenge of providing you with the support you need

- Inadvertently doing or saying invalidating or hurtful things and feeling confused about the "right" or most effective thing to do or say

- Tending to treat you as if you are your disorder, or as if you'll always do the same things or feel the same way as you have in the past

Fear and Worry

One of the most common experiences among the loved ones we've worked with is a painful cycle of fear, worry, and guilt. Often the fear grows out of concerns about the safety of the person with BPD and is amplified when certain problems occur, such as suicide attempts, self-harm, drug or alcohol use, reckless behaviors, or difficulties with self-care. For parents in particular, the idea of a child committing suicide or attempting to do so is both terrifying and heartbreaking. As a result, parents often spend a lot of time living in fear and worrying about what might happen. That's not to say that if you've done these things, you are to blame for your loved ones' worries and fears, or that you're a burden on them. If they were in your shoes, experiencing the kind of pain you experience, they would probably be doing the same things. Furthermore, although your loved ones' fears are indeed understandable, natural reactions to overwhelming situations, they often create more problems.

One problem with fear and worry is that when they're in the driver's seat, your loved ones will actually become less effective at supporting you. Fear makes people's attention narrow and focus on any signs that a threatening event might occur. This is known as hypervigilance. With hypervigilance, people are alert to any signs of danger and will go to great lengths to prevent it. In effect, they get tunnel vision and can't see the bigger picture. When your loved ones feel this way, your relationship can suffer in several ways:

- Because they're so focused on maintaining your safety, they might not be able to listen to you or give you the help and support you need.

- They might do whatever you want them to do and push themselves to be there for you all the time, even though this burns them out, resulting in stress and resentment.

- They might smother you with attention or treat you as if you're fragile and unable to cope or independently do things for yourself.

- They might avoid confrontation or bringing things up that would be important to talk about.

- They might go through cycles of being there for you in a very intense way and then withdrawing, leaving you feeling rejected or abandoned.

Guilt

Guilt is another common reaction, particularly among parents. They might wonder whether they're at least partly to blame for your mental health difficulties. Your parents may mentally replay events from your childhood again and again, looking for things they might have done that put you on the path to your current difficulties. And indeed, in some cases, parents' or caregivers' actions may have played an important role in the development of BPD.

The problem is that many people don't know how to deal with guilt effectively. Some people even end up feeling angry or resentful of the person they feel guilty toward. Perhaps you've experienced this yourself. You may have done or said something and feel guilty about it, but if the other person brings it up, you get angry with her or him for mentioning it and "making you feel guilty." This is a pretty common cycle of events, and it has negative effects on relationships.

Another problem with guilt is that it's a very painful emotion. Therefore, if your loved ones feel guilty, they might seek to avoid that emotion at all costs. You may miss the opportunity to really talk with them about how their actions have (or haven't) affected you if they avoid the topic or become so distressed that they end the conversation before the two of you reach any resolution or closure. Because guilt is so painful, your loved ones might also go to great lengths to absolve themselves of whatever they feel guilty about, perhaps by apologizing excessively, making repeated attempts to repair the relationship when doing so is unnecessary, and so on.

The bottom line is that guilt is a very common experience among family members, partners, and friends of people with mental health problems (not just BPD). It's important to be aware of this so you have a better understanding of what your loved ones might be going through and what might be motivating some of their actions.

EFFECTIVE COMMUNICATION WITH LOVED ONES

Now that we've discussed some of the challenges that can arise with loved ones, let's look at solutions. With relationship issues, the best place to start is usually with communication. To help ease communications about your BPD with loved ones, several skills and strategies will be immensely helpful:

- Come up with ground rules that work for you.

- Be clear and direct about your needs.

- Keep the relationship in mind.

- Manage conflict effectively.

Come Up with Ground Rules

A good starting point in navigating interactions with loved ones is to come up with ground rules. When others don't know what's okay to bring up or how best to address a topic, their uncertainty can get in the way of effective communication. They may avoid topics that would be helpful to discuss, or they may bring up difficult topics suddenly or abruptly. One way around this is to come up with some ground rules ahead of time, clarifying what will work best for you in your recovery and what won't work, and then share these ground rules with your loved ones. Here are some ideas on ground rules you may wish to establish:

Crises, emergencies, and suicide risk. Work with loved ones to come up with a clear game plan on how they can respond and help during crises. Consider whether it's acceptable for them to contact your treatment provider if they feel it's warranted or how they might ensure that you go to the hospital if you're at very high risk. Tell your loved ones how they can best help you when you're in a crisis and your emotions are overwhelming, such as by reminding you of important coping skills, staying close by, helping to distract you with activities, going somewhere for a walk or drive, encouraging you to exercise, and so on. (Chapter 8, on lifestyle approaches to support mental health, will give you more information on these types of strategies.)

Keeping up with medications, treatment, or both. Because your loved ones probably have a strong investment in your well-being, they may feel distressed if it seems that you aren't following through with your therapy or medications. Be sure to establish how involved you want them to be in supporting your treatment efforts and how independent you want to be in this area. Be specific about how they should handle any apparent lapses. Do you want them to remind you of things or ask whether you've taken your medication, or would you prefer that you initiate any conversations on this topic?

Work. Another area where loved ones can become quite concerned and involved, for better or worse, is work. If you're having trouble getting work or maintaining employment, or if you're struggling at work, you may want to discuss what level of involvement of your loved ones is acceptable to you. How would you like them to approach this topic, or would you prefer that they remain uninvolved? Do you want them to check in with you about how work or a job search is going or offer advice or opinions?

Relationships. Considerations around ground rules for relationship issues are similar to those regarding work. Think about what's acceptable to you in terms of involvement in your other relationships, friendships, intimate relationships, and so on. Parents or caregivers, in particular, can become quite worried and possibly overinvolved if you're in a close relationship with someone they perceive as being not good for you.

Another part of coming up with ground rules is to make deals with loved ones ahead of time. There are two important deals that we suggest you consider making. First, make a deal that, if you're seeking some kind of support, you'll be explicit about what kind of support you need or want. Have you ever had the experience where a conversation gets completely derailed because you start talking about an upsetting event and the other person jumps in with advice and suggestions, when you really just wanted someone to listen and understand? On the other hand, sometimes you might want advice and suggestions, and the person only listens and offers sympathy.

In order to get your needs met, let others know up front exactly what you're looking for. For example, you might say, "I've had the worst day ever at work, and eventually I'm going to want your help in figuring out how to change things. But right now, I just need your support and to feel understood." You can also make a deal that, if you forget to be clear about what kind of support you want, your loved one will ask you what you need before the conversation gets started—or at least before it gets off track.

A second important deal to make is that each person will allow the other to take a time-out if the conversation gets too heated and is headed in unproductive or unhelpful directions. So often, two well-intentioned people enter a conversation only to leave it demoralized, distressed, or even in crisis. How does this happen? Often the conversation gets heated and triggers overwhelming emotions for one or both people. When emotions are that high, it's difficult to be skillful in the conversation. The value of this particular deal is that both of you get a chance to take a breather and regulate or manage emotions so you can return to the conversation in a calmer state of mind.

It's critical that both parties agree to the strategy of taking time-outs ahead of time. Sometimes one person might want to keep talking even though the other person is getting really upset. If you're the one getting upset, it may be hard to take a time-out if you haven't established a ground rule about this in advance. If you try to leave the conversation or the room, the other person might follow you or continue to try to engage you in the discussion. Time-outs should be brief, ideally between ten minutes and an hour, and both parties must agree to return to the conversation afterward so the issue can actually be resolved.

Be Clear about Your Needs

As indicated in the first "deal" we outlined above, it's important to communicate your needs clearly. In DBT, clients learn skills for effectively asking for what they need; in essence, these skills involve being clear and direct. We'll walk you through the steps involved in being clear about your needs with an imaginary scenario, and then you can apply this approach to situations in your own life.

Let's say the situation is that you've been out of work for a while, in part due to mental health challenges. You feel ashamed of not working, but you're also scared and overwhelmed at the prospect of looking for a job, filling out applications, doing interviews, and so on. Let's also say that your partner keeps asking you about your job search, and in response, you feel even more overwhelmed and ashamed. Here's an outline of how you can clearly state your needs, based on the interpersonal effectiveness skills in DBT (Linehan 1993b):

1. **Describe the situation.** Start by telling the person what's going on. Be clear and concise, and leave out any criticism, judgments, or inflammatory statements about the other person. Avoid extreme terms, such as "bad," "should" or "shouldn't," "jerk," "always," "never," and so on. Here's an example: "I've been really stressed-out because I'm out of work and scared of applying and going through interviews."

2. **Describe and express how you feel.** Focus on your emotions, and make sure you own your emotions by using "I" statements. A formula that a lot of people use in couples therapy is "I feel X when you do [or say] Y." Owning your feelings, rather than making it seem like they're entirely the other person's fault, will help the other person be less defensive and more receptive to what you have to say— for example, "When you ask me how the job search is going, I feel overwhelmed, anxious, and a little ashamed that I'm not working."

3. **Tell the person what you need or want.** Be clear about exactly what you need or want from the other person. You might think that simply saying, "I want more respect" or "Please be sensitive to how I feel" should be enough. However, such requests are so vague that people often can't understand exactly what you need and want. Make sure you frame your request in terms of specific actions or

behaviors rather than in broad ideas or concepts—for example, "If you could ask me a little less often or let me take a break or change the topic when I don't feel up to talking about it, I'd feel a lot better, and I might feel less frightened about looking for a job."

Keep the Relationship in Mind

When seeking the support you need, it's important to think through how your interactions with loved ones might affect the relationship over the long run. One consideration has to do with how you ask for support. We recommend that you follow the old adage "You can catch more flies with honey than with vinegar." People are more likely to support you and do so gladly if you ask for what you want or need in a gentle but clear manner than if you express judgments or criticisms. Sometimes you might feel like the only way to get your message across is to yell, scream, threaten, or even hurt yourself. And in some cases, this may actually be true in the short term. The problem is that these types of behaviors generally interfere with relationships in the long run.

It's also important to think through whether you're going to extremes regarding requests for support. One extreme would be to never ask for what you want or need, in which case you're likely to end up feeling either resentful that others aren't supporting you or unimportant (because you aren't treating your needs as important). The other extreme would be always asking for what you need, whenever you need it. This, too, can strain relationships, as others may feel they have to provide more support than they can reasonably manage, perhaps leading to burnout or resentment on their part. Think about where you fall on the continuum between never asking for what you need versus always asking for what you need or even demanding it. Try to edge a little closer to what is referred to in DBT as the "middle path" (Linehan 1993a, 1993b), seeking the support you need but remaining aware that other people have limits regarding what they are able or willing to provide. If you keep these two considerations in mind and do your best to walk the middle path in terms of when, how often, and how you seek support, you'll probably find that your relationships benefit and you get your needs met.

Manage Conflict Effectively

From time to time, you might find that even when both people involved in the conversation have the best of intentions, the interaction becomes heated. If you've agreed on the strategy of taking time-outs when needed, that will help. But you also need to know what to do once you're in the middle of a heated discussion or conflict with a loved one.

First, perhaps the most important thing to do is to step back in your mind, stop talking, and observe your emotions. Start by just noticing how you're feeling. Are you hurt, angry, frustrated, or feeling rejected? Try your best to accept your emotions for what they are; there's probably a very good reason you feel this way. Then take a deep breath, relax your posture and muscles, and try to become a bit more centered. Pay attention to your feelings and, for just a moment, don't act on them.

Second, do your best to practice damage control (we'll discuss this further in the next chapter). In other words, try not to make things worse. If you've said hurtful things, try your best to stop and not say anything until you can offer something effective, skillful, or kind. Another way to avoid making things worse is to lower the volume or tone of your voice, particularly if the conversation has escalated to shouting. Assume a nonthreatening, relaxed posture and speak more calmly, softly, and quietly (just be careful to avoid doing so in a patronizing manner). When people raise their voices at the same time, each person's agitation tends to increase exponentially in response to the other person's tone of voice, demeanor, and posture. Dialing down your intensity should help reduce the other person's intensity as well.

Third, don't respond to attacks or criticisms unless absolutely necessary. If things have become so heated that the other person is insulting or verbally attacking you, sometimes the most effective thing to do is simply ignore the criticism. This is one of the interpersonal effectiveness skills in DBT, where it's called ignoring attacks (Linehan 1993b). Simply dodge any attacks that come your way; don't give them the time of day. Responding to attacks often invites more attacks or leads to debates and long lists of each other's flaws, like whether you wash the dishes, do the laundry, get out of bed on time, and so on. This upsets both parties, and it's also a waste of time. Just as ignoring a child who's throwing a tantrum will eventually teach the child not to do this, ignoring people who verbally attack you can teach them to stop.

However, if you're at risk of physical violence from a loved one—or anyone—your top priority must be your own safety. If this is a factor in your living situation, make sure you have a backup safety plan: arrange for someplace safe to go and for someone who can help you, and be aware of when or whether you might need to call for help, such as calling the police.

MOVING FORWARD

BPD presents challenges both for you and for your loved ones. Some of the most common effects on loved ones are confusion, fear, worry, and guilt. Other challenges include difficulties in knowing how much or how little to help, when to bring up certain topics, and how to handle emergencies. Your loved ones may not know how to navigate these issues in a way that works for each of you. Perhaps the most helpful thing you can do is communicate your needs clearly. Also try the other strategies described in this chapter, such as setting ground rules, keeping the relationship in mind, and managing conflict effectively. If you practice these skills regularly, we're confident that you'll start to notice some positive changes in your relationships.

In the next chapter, we'll discuss techniques that can help you tolerate and manage overwhelming emotions. This will be beneficial in and of itself, and it may also help you navigate relationships and difficult communications with loved ones more effectively.

CHAPTER 7

Learning to Manage
Overwhelming
Emotions

If you have BPD, you're probably no stranger to strong, overwhelming emotions. You may often feel swept up in huge waves of emotion and unsure of what to do to get yourself back in control again. Although this type of intense emotional experience can be overwhelming, painful, and confusing, your emotions themselves are not the problem. There's nothing inherently wrong with being an emotional person. Some of the most interesting people we know are quite emotional. Indeed, many celebrities and highly successful people are known to be very emotional and passionate, such as Gordon Ramsay (most famous for the series *Hell's Kitchen*), the late Steve Jobs (of Apple), Oprah Winfrey, and even Marsha Linehan (who developed DBT).

Although there's nothing inherently wrong with strong emotions, they can sometimes steer you in directions you don't want to go. Perhaps strong emotions such as anger, sadness, or shame have led you to do things you later regretted, such as yelling at others, harming yourself, using drugs, attempting suicide, or taking risks. This can make it seem as if strong emotions are useless troublemakers and you'd be better off without them. We know, however, that you don't have to get rid of these emotions to have a good life. You can have strong emotions and still stay on course if you learn how to tolerate and manage them. Therefore, in this chapter, we'll give you some pointers on how to manage strong emotions so you can keep moving forward in directions that are important to you.

UNDERSTANDING EMOTIONS

Although your emotions may sometimes seem confusing, painful, and unnecessary, emotions are actually very important for survival and for good relationships with others. Think of your emotions as being like a complex weather station, registering the air temperature, barometric pressure, wind speed, and so on, and communicating these important facts to whomever needs to know them. In a similar way, an emotional response, consisting of changes in your brain (neurochemical activity) and body (heart rate, perspiration, muscle tension, urges to do things), can tell you that something is happening that you might need to pay attention to. Perhaps a storm is on the horizon, or maybe a sunny day is forecast. Fear, for example, might alert you to danger, whereas anger might tell you that you have been hurt or wronged in some way.

Emotions also make you feel like doing things, triggering action urges, as they are called in DBT (Linehan 1993b). When you're afraid, you might feel like escaping your current situation. When you're angry, you might feel like fighting or protecting yourself. Happiness and love might make you want to be closer to another person.

Emotions can help you act wisely and do things you need to do. However, they can also lead you astray when they're exceptionally intense or overwhelming, or when they're false alarms, such as feeling afraid in the absence of any real danger. It can also be very hard for some people with BPD to tolerate specific emotions, such as shame or sadness. And when you have a hard time tolerating your emotions, you might resort to unhealthy coping strategies to get rid of them or reduce their intensity, such as self-harm, drug use, and suicidal behavior. The good news is, several skills, ideally used in a stepwise way, can help you learn to tolerate your emotions and manage them more effectively (Linehan 1993b):

1. Observing and labeling emotions

2. Doing damage control

3. Calming the storm

1. OBSERVE AND LABEL YOUR EMOTIONS

The first step in managing emotions and learning to tolerate them is to take a step back in your mind and try to get a good look at what you're feeling. By taking the time to figure out how you're feeling before you act, instead of immediately acting on your emotions or reacting to the situation, you give yourself the opportunity to respond more wisely. This can help you avoid the common pitfalls of acting on emotions without thinking. To use this skill, take a quick breather the next time you feel a moderate to strong emotion, following these steps:

1. **Stop whatever you're doing.** The best way to avoid trouble when you're highly emotional is to begin by doing nothing at all. If you're talking with someone and you're so upset that you can't say anything effective, stop talking for a moment. If you're walking somewhere and you're hit with a strong emotion, take a moment to sit on a bench or at least walk more slowly.

2. **Take a few deep breaths.** Try to breathe from your abdomen and not your chest. Abdominal breathing brings more air deeper into your lungs and creates a good ratio of oxygen to carbon dioxide in your blood. This will directly reduce tension and anxiety.

3. **Relax your muscles and any tension in your body.** Try to get yourself into a calm, relaxed posture. It's amazing how the body communicates with the brain. If you allow

your body to relax in the face of painful emotions, your brain will start to get the signal that you're safe. If you tense up, your brain starts to prepare you for drastic action—exactly what you probably don't want to do when experiencing overwhelming emotions.

Along with having more intense emotions, people with BPD may be more likely to experience conflicting emotions (both positive emotions, such as happiness, and negative emotions, such as sadness) at close to the same time (Ebner-Priemer et al. 2008). This can make emotions both frightening and confusing. Simply labeling your emotions (such as saying to yourself, I'm feeling sad or I'm feeling angry), however, may make them feel more manageable, take the edge off these feelings, and reduce emotional arousal (Lieberman et al. 2007).

So, how do you go about figuring out what you're feeling and putting a label on your emotions? We suggest that you begin by doing a body scan, mainly because your body is where you experience emotions. The body scan involves paying attention to the sensations you feel physically, in your body, when you experience a strong emotion. Start with your feet and pay close attention to whatever you feel in your feet. For example, they might feel hot, cool, tense, achy, or neutral. After paying attention to your feet, move up sequentially to your ankles, calves, legs, abdomen, chest, hands, arms, shoulders, neck, and head. As you attend to each area of your body, try to notice any sensations that might be coming along with your emotion. Try to localize where you're feeling your emotion physically, and describe the sensations to yourself. For example, if you're feeling angry, perhaps you'd say, *My chest feels tight, my jaw is tense, my heart is pounding, my hands feel hot, and my brow is furrowed.* If you're feeling sad, you might say, *I feel tension behind my eyes, my eyes are teary, my voice is quavering, my arms and legs feel heavy, and I feel emptiness and a sinking sensation in my stomach.*

You might notice that you're experiencing several different emotions, such as anger, sadness, shame, and so on. If so, do your best to sort out what you're feeling and perhaps focus on the emotion that's hardest to tolerate or manage. Finally, ask yourself how intense or strong your emotions are. You may find it helpful to use a scale, such as one from 0 (no emotion at all) to 100 (unbelievably intense).

To most effectively sort out and label your emotions, we recommend using a four-column worksheet like the one that follows, a prontable version of which is available for download at www.newharbinger.com/27060. In the Emotions column, write down any emotion you're feeling. In the Sensations column, describe the physical sensations associated with each emotion. In the Urges column, describe any action impulses—in other words, what you feel like doing in response to the emotion. Finally, in the Intensity column, rate how strong the emotion is using a scale from 0 to 100.

Emotion What emotion are you feeling?	Sensations What sensations do you feel?	Urges What do you feel like doing?	Intensity How strong is the emotion? (0-100)

2. DO DAMAGE CONTROL

The next step in managing strong emotions is damage control; in other words, not making things worse. In DBT, the distress tolerance skills start off with a set of strategies to help you with damage control (Linehan 1993b). The idea is that intense emotions are challenging enough to manage on their own without adding any additional suffering by doing something you'll later regret.

You're probably familiar with some of the ways you can make things worse when you're experiencing an intense emotion. When you feel extremely emotional, it's natural to look for a way to escape painful feelings. Unfortunately, with BPD, escape strategies often involve behaviors that are harmful to yourself or others, such as self-injury, other self-destructive actions, yelling, or throwing things at others. Other ways of escaping emotional pain might involve isolating yourself, avoiding work or chores, or skipping out of important responsibilities at home, school, or work. Think about things you've done in the past when you experienced overwhelming emotions and identify which made your situation worse, either in the short term or the long term, then do your best to avoid doing them in the future. Of course, this is easier said than done, so in the following sections we'll describe some strategies that may help.

Avoid Doing Anything

Sit on your hands—literally. Avoid moving or doing or saying anything until you can do or say something that's either wise or in your best interests. Simply stop doing anything and everything until you can do something that will make things better—or at least not worse.

Get Support

You may benefit from having a support person around to help you avoid certain behaviors, such as drinking, using drugs, self-harming, or any other damaging behaviors you're drawn to do when you're very upset. If you use this strategy, make sure you choose someone who is understanding and will actually support you. When you're already overwhelmed, the last thing you need is conflict with your support person.

Go to a Safe Environment

Go someplace where it would be hard to do anything self-destructive, such as a mall, coffee shop, grocery store, recreation center, gym, or park. Beyond helping you with damage control, sometimes simply getting out of the place in which you're feeling pain and misery can shift your mood and thinking in another direction.

Use Distraction Strategies

Another way to avoid making things worse is to distract yourself and get your mind off whatever is bothering you (Linehan 1993b). In fact, many of the self-destructive things people do when they're upset, such as self-harm, help in the moment by providing a distraction from emotional pain. Of course, we recommend that if you use distraction, you choose positive activities that enhance your well-being. We also recommend that you use this strategy sparingly and only when truly needed. After all, you don't want to end up distracting your life away!

To distract yourself, you need to do something that gets your mind busy—so busy that you don't have much room to think about or dwell on what's upsetting you. Here are some suggestions for ways to distract yourself:

- **Get your mind working.** Give your mind something else to focus on other than what's upsetting you. Do a crossword or Sudoku puzzle; play a game on your smartphone or computer; focus your attention on schoolwork, balancing your checkbook, or some other demanding mental task; or count backward from 663 by threes until you reach zero. Any task that makes your mind work should help.

- **Get active.** Throw yourself into some kind of engaging activity. Beyond distracting you from whatever is bothering you, doing a different activity might take the edge off your emotions or shift your mood. Particularly helpful activities include going for a walk; playing or practicing sports, martial arts, or yoga; working out; talking with someone (about something other than what's bothering you); checking out an interesting area of your town that you don't normally visit; watching a stimulating TV show or movie; helping other people or animals; or cleaning or doing housework, perhaps while listening to your favorite music (some of these suggestions come from Marsha Linehan's *Skills Training Manual for Treating Borderline Personality Disorder*; Linehan 1993b).

3. CALM THE STORM

Another important step in learning to manage your emotions involves doing things that will help you calm your mind and regulate your emotions. Many people with BPD never learned how to regulate intense emotions, because the people around them were invalidating, didn't have such intense emotions, or didn't know how to regulate intense emotions themselves. Therefore, don't worry if some of the skills below don't come naturally to you at first; the more you practice them, the more natural they will feel.

Self-Soothing

Self-soothing involves using the power of your five senses to soothe and calm your mind and body (Linehan 1993b). To practice this skill, come up with a list of as many things as you can think of that you find calming or soothing in some way, and that involve your five senses. Here are some suggestions:

- **Vision.** Look at a beautiful painting or pictures of a person or place you love; watch children or pets play in a park; look at flowers or trees; watch a sunset;

watch a television show about nature; or look at photos on your computer or smartphone.

- **Hearing.** Listen to music (some people find loud heavy metal soothing, so it doesn't have to be classical or new age music—any music that's soothing to you will work); listen to a cat purring on your lap or birds chirping; or sit outside and just pay attention to all the sounds you hear.

- **Smell.** Use aromatherapy candles; walk into a flower shop; smell a fresh cup of coffee or coffee beans; walk into a bakery; or put on your favorite perfume or cologne.

- **Taste.** Drink a fresh cup of decaffeinated coffee or tea; eat a small amount of your favorite comfort food; suck on a mint or candy; or eat an ice cream cone.

- **Touch.** Put freshly laundered sheets on your bed; stroke an animal; wear a soft fabric; get a massage or do self-massage; or hug someone close to you.

We're confident that some of these strategies will work very well for you. We've made these pages available in printable form at www.newharbinger.com/27060 so that you can put them up wherever you practice them as a reminder. However, to use this skill to your best advantage, there are three tricks to keep in mind: First, because self-soothing strategies can become less effective over time, keep some backup ideas in mind and also be willing to try new things. Second, pay very close attention to your experience while self-soothing; in other words, tune in and be mindful of your sensory experience. Third, while engaged in self-soothing, try to ignore any thoughts that these activities are a waste of time or that you don't deserve to be taking care of yourself. If and when these thoughts arise, simply notice them and then bring your attention back to the soothing activity, allowing the thoughts to pass through your mind.

Physical Activities

Sometimes the best way to calm the storm is to do something physical that directly affects the physiological aspects of your emotional arousal. What happens to your body can profoundly affect your mood. Effective and nonharmful physical approaches to managing emotions include changing your body temperature, doing an activity that gets your heart pumping, or doing something that calms or relaxes your body. We are indebted to Marsha Linehan (Linehan, forthcoming) for many of the suggestions below.

CHANGE YOUR BODY TEMPERATURE

Take a warm, soothing bath, above lukewarm but not too hot. (A hot bath can actually raise your heart rate.) Soak your feet in warm water with a few drops of lavender essential oil or another calming aromatherapy oil. Go outside into the bracing cold air on a winter's day, or stand in the rain for a little while. Sit outdoors and feel the heat of the sun on your face. Wrap a couple of packs of ice in a thin towel and place them gently on your face, or put cold, wet washcloths on your face. Fill a large bowl with cold water and ice and dunk your face into the ice water a few times, for about five to ten seconds each time (while holding your breath, of course). All of these activities will change your heart rate, which may help decrease emotional arousal and calm your body.

ENGAGE IN PHYSICAL EXERCISE

Physical exercise can be one of the best ways to change your emotional state and make things feel more bearable. If you're experiencing overwhelming emotions, it's likely that your sympathetic nervous system, responsible for the fight-or-flight response, is strongly activated. Although exercise has some of the same effects on your body, elevating your heart rate and increasing your body temperature, the aftereffects of exercise are almost the exact opposite, with most physiological systems slowing down, leaving your body more relaxed than it was before you started exercising.

Another benefit of exercise is that, if you're experiencing a high-energy type of emotion, such as anger, anxiety, or agitation, your brain may attribute your body's revved-up state to exercising, rather than emotional distress. In essence, exercise can trick your brain into thinking that the reason you're feeling amped up is because you're exercising, not because you're emotionally distressed. When using this skill, try to choose some form of exercise that's fairly intense for you, whatever your fitness level might be. This could include running, jogging, walking up and down stairs, doing push-ups or sit-ups, or even more calming types of exercise, such as yoga or Pilates. You may notice more benefits if you're able

115

to do the exercise outside in the fresh air or if the activity is fun or enjoyable for you, in addition to being physically demanding.

USE RELAXATION STRATEGIES

There are many different relaxation strategies, but most involve using the power of your body and breath to regulate your emotions. An excellent relaxation strategy that focuses on the body is *progressive muscle relaxation* (PMR). It involves systematically tensing and relaxing muscles throughout your body, usually starting with your toes and working your way up to your face, neck, and head. As you focus on each muscle group, tense your muscles with approximately 75 percent of your strength, hold the tension for several seconds, and then relax. Pay close attention to how the muscles feel both while you're tensing them and when you relax. PMR can help you be more aware of the difference between muscular tension and relaxation, allowing you to notice physical tension and relax more easily. You can find detailed instructions for PMR on the Internet. It takes some practice, so try it out on a daily basis for the next week or two, and then give it a try the next time you feel emotionally overwhelmed.

In terms of the breath, two different types of breathing can be tremendously helpful in regulating the emotional systems of your body and brain. One is *diaphragmatic breathing*. To practice diaphragmatic breathing, sit in a relaxed but upright position, with your shoulders back, and put one hand on your chest and the other on your midbelly region, around your diaphragm (located near the bottom of your ribs). Slowly draw air into your lungs by expanding your abdomen, not your chest, and when you exhale, do so slowly and evenly, gently pushing the air out with your abdomen. Diaphragmatic or abdominal breathing provides a much better balance of oxygen to carbon dioxide in the blood than shallow, chest breathing, which is associated with anxiety, tension, and panic.

The second type of breathing that can be helpful is *paced breathing*. To do paced breathing, follow the instructions for diaphragmatic breathing, but when you breathe in, count quietly to yourself ("one, two, three") at a pace of about one second per count. When you breathe out, count quietly to yourself again. Try to slowly increase the count. It's most important to extend the exhalation, rather than the inhalation, so focus on slowing your out-breath in particular. This will activate your body's natural relaxation system (the parasympathetic nervous system) and reduce your heart rate and blood pressure.

Express Yourself

Another way to manage overwhelming emotions is to express them. This doesn't mean it's helpful to spend a lot of time venting about whatever you're upset about. However, expressing how you feel, either to yourself or to others, can be like opening a release valve on your emotions and may help ease your suffering a bit. There are many ways to express your emotions, including seeking out a caring, supportive listener and talking about what's going on and how you feel; writing in a journal or diary; expressing your emotions through art or music; or simply saying how you feel to yourself, either out loud or in your mind.

BORDERLINE PERSONALITY DISORDER

With sadness in particular, another way to express your emotions is to allow yourself to cry. Some of the people we've worked with are afraid to cry, even when they're alone. As a result, they stifle themselves and never experience the benefits of crying, which include the release of stress hormones through tears, the physical relief that often follows crying, and the acknowledgment to yourself that you're having a hard time, which can be self-validating. If you feel like crying, we suggest that you pay mindful attention to your experience and let the crying run its course. Don't try to either amplify or stifle the experience. Just let it happen, and when the urge to cry passes, let it pass. Pay attention to how you feel both before and after crying to see whether it has been helpful. As strange as it might sound, effective crying can be a worthwhile skill to master.

PREVENTING OVERWHELMING EMOTIONS

As you become more familiar with emotions and what's likely to trigger them, sometimes you may be able to prevent them from becoming overwhelming. Try to predict strong emotional responses ahead of time and then head them off at the pass. Although we don't have the space to cover all of the ways for you to do this, we recommend that you try the following strategies for what in DBT is called coping ahead of time:

- When you're in a relatively calm state of mind, sit down and trace out some of the factors in life that

118

really trigger you or make you miserable. Then try to find solutions for at least some of them.

- Proactively plan ahead for how you might cope with upcoming sources of stress or difficult situations.

- Seek help from your therapist or mental health provider to determine how to avert crises before they even happen.

- Slowly make positive changes in your life that reduce your vulnerability to overwhelming emotions by working on your self-care, improving your relationships with others, and spending more time doing things that you value, enjoy, and find meaningful (Linehan 1993b).

MOVING FORWARD

This chapter focused on ways to survive and manage overwhelming emotions. We reviewed three important steps to take when you're feeling overwhelmed emotionally: observing and labeling your emotions, doing damage control, and calming the storm. We recommend that you practice all of these skills when things are relatively calm; that way you'll be much better prepared to use them when emotional storms hit. In the next chapter, we'll look at how you can create and maintain a lifestyle that supports physical and mental health, including skills for doing the things that matter to you and building a meaningful life for yourself.

CHAPTER 8

DEVELOPING A LIFESTYLE THAT SUPPORTS MENTAL HEALTH

In the previous chapter, we discussed several skills that may help you manage or cope with emotions that are intense or unpleasant. Knowing what to do when strong emotions put you at risk for doing something impulsive is incredibly important to your recovery and could very well help you avoid some of the hazards of BPD. However, knowing what to do in crisis situations is just one piece of the puzzle. It's just as important to use skills on a daily basis to create and maintain a healthy lifestyle overall—a lifestyle that supports your mental health and well-being. Doing so can make it easier to use some of the healthy coping strategies we've already taught you in this book, and can even prevent some crises from occurring.

IDENTIFYING SOURCES OF STRESS

Unfortunately, stress is unavoidable; it's a part of life for everyone. Stress can also have a major impact on people's mental health and emotional well-being. So, what is stress exactly? This may come as a surprise to you, but the term "stress" doesn't actually refer to a particular type of experience or situation; it refers to the response your body has when you are faced with circumstances that force you to act, change, or adjust to your environment. Stress has a purpose: it tells us that the body's resources are being taxed or used up in some way.

Imagine that your body is a car. As you probably know, there are some very powerful cars out there that can get from point A to point B relatively quickly. However, let's say that you're moving to a new home. You might start out slow, loading up your car with a few small boxes. Chances are that this won't have much impact on your car's performance. You probably won't notice any difference in how the car handles or its ability to get up to speed. Now let's say that you decide to start loading up your car with heavier items from your home. You might notice how the car's frame starts to sink under the weight. You might notice that the car is harder to maneuver or strains to maintain its speed when going up steep hills. Basically, the more stress you put on the car, the more difficulty it will have performing well.

This is what happens when people experience stress. Stress weighs us down and affects the body's ability to perform everyday functions. It can affect our appetite, sleep, thoughts, and emotions. Just like cars, human beings have only a limited amount of resources available to deal with all the demands of daily life. The more situations we encounter that use up these resources, the more stressed-out, tense, or depleted we will feel and the less effective we become in managing those situations. You might also notice that you have fewer resources available to manage your emotions and that the more stressed-out you are, the more intense and overwhelming your emotions become.

The good news is that even though stress is unavoidable, there are steps you can take to reduce its impact on your life. The first step is to identify the types of events or situations that are stressful for you. At the beginning of each week, take some time to write down the sources of stress you expect to encounter during the week, such as an exam, a performance review at work, a family reunion, a doctor's appointment you are worried about, or a hectic work schedule. Although this won't prevent these stressful situations from occurring, it will make you more aware of your potential sources of stress and their impact on your mental and physical health.

Knowing that these situations are on your horizon can also help you prepare for them in advance. For example, if you see that you are facing a particularly stressful week, you might want to schedule some time to do something relaxing, such as getting a massage or seeing a movie. If you have a lot that you need to accomplish during the week, you may want to come up with a schedule to help keep you organized and on track. Being aware of upcoming sources of stress can go a long way in reducing their impact on your emotional health.

TAKING CARE OF YOUR BODY

Your physical health and the overall state of your body can have a major impact on your ability to manage your emotions and cope with crises successfully. People's emotions, thoughts, and bodies are all interconnected and influence one another. If your body is in poor shape, this will probably trickle down to your emotions and thoughts. For example, think of a time when you didn't get much sleep or didn't sleep well. How did you feel the next day? You may have noticed that you felt more on edge or that your emotions seemed more intense. You might have noticed that you were more likely to react to things that happened or things people said, including things that normally wouldn't bother you. You may also have noticed that you felt down and depressed or had difficulty focusing on or enjoying positive or fun activities in your day.

Because how you treat your body can have a major impact on how you feel, anything you can do to take care of yourself physically, including getting enough sleep, watching what you eat, taking care of your body when you are ill, and limiting your alcohol and drug intake, will have benefits for your mental health (Linehan 1993b). Many of the skills discussed in the following sections come from Dr. Marsha Linehan's *Skills Training Manual for Treating Borderline Personality Disorder* (1993b).

Maintaining a Balanced Diet

One way to improve and maintain your day-to-day emotional health is to eat nutritious food and establish healthy eating habits (Linehan 1993b). Your body needs a variety of nutrients to live and to function at its best, so maintaining a healthy diet will ensure you have the fuel and building blocks your body needs. It's also important to eat regularly throughout the day, spacing out your meals and snacks. If you eat just one or two big meals during the day, you might get a burst of energy, but you will probably crash soon afterward. Eating smaller meals and snacks more frequently will give you a consistent supply of energy throughout your day. A common recommendation is to eat three meals and two snacks per day.

Be sure to eat healthy quantities and types of foods as well. Junk food, or any food high in sugar or fat, might give you an initial boost of energy, but the energy it provides is short-lived. It's healthier to eat plenty of fruits, vegetables, whole grains, and proteins. This doesn't mean that you can't sometimes indulge in a rich dessert or your favorite junk food. Any food can be part of a healthy diet as long as it's eaten in moderation. The goal is not to eat only certain foods and avoid others, but to maintain a balanced diet across all food groups. If you are unsure about what to eat or how to maintain a well-balanced, healthy diet, you may want to talk with your physician, a nutritionist, or a dietician. You could also consult the websites of the US Food and Drug Administration and Health Canada, both of which contain dietary guidelines and food and nutrition information.

Developing Good Sleep Habits

Just as your body needs the right nutrients to run well, it also needs enough sleep (Linehan 1993b). When you don't get enough sleep, it's like starting off your day without a full tank of gas. Now, there may be some days when you only need half a tank of gas to get where you're going, so starting out a bit low on fuel isn't as much of a problem. But what about those days that resemble long road trips, when you have a lot of distance to cover and many places to go? Starting off without a full tank of gas on days like those might be more of a problem. It could leave you running on fumes partway through the day. And, as you've probably experienced, this will have a major impact on how you feel and your ability to manage any stressors that come your way.

You may be thinking that getting enough sleep is easier said than done. If so, you are absolutely right. Developing healthy sleeping patterns is not an easy thing to do, especially if you've been having difficulties sleeping for a while. Fortunately, there are several steps you can take to develop better sleep habits and improve your sleep (Bourne 1995; Perlis et al. 2008); we've collected them in the following list, a printable version of which is available online at www.newharbinger.com/27060.

- Keep a regular sleep schedule. Choose a consistent time to go to bed each night and get up each morning. Stick to this schedule even if you don't feel ready to go to bed or feel too tired to get up. This will help your body establish a good sleep-wake cycle.

- Avoid taking naps during the day, as this can greatly impair your ability to fall asleep at night.

- Don't go to bed hungry, but don't eat right before you go to bed either. Try to eat a few hours before your bedtime to give your body some time to digest the meal before you go to bed.

- If you exercise, try to exercise in the morning or during the day. It's best to avoid exercising within six hours of your bedtime. Exercising right before bed can rev your body up and make it more difficult to fall asleep.

- Limit the amount of caffeine you consume during the day. If you struggle to fall asleep at night, or if you know you are sensitive to caffeine, you may want to avoid caffeine completely after lunchtime, including foods that contain caffeine, such as chocolate. Caffeine sticks around in the body for a long time. In fact, it can take five to six hours for the body to process half the caffeine from a cup of coffee.

- Limit your intake of nicotine, particularly close to bedtime. Although some people think smoking relaxes them, the relaxation they experience is just a reduction in their cravings for nicotine. Smoking doesn't actually do anything to help with stress. In fact, nicotine is a stimulant. Therefore, the more you smoke during the day, the harder it may be for you to fall asleep at night, especially if you smoke right before bed. For this reason, try to avoid having a cigarette right before bedtime.

- Similarly, limit the amount of alcohol you consume and avoid consuming alcohol within six hours of your bedtime. Like nicotine, alcohol can be a stimulant, particularly shortly after it is consumed. Therefore, drinking too much alcohol (especially right before bedtime) can rev up your body. Drinking more than moderate amounts of alcohol can also interfere with the quality of your sleep, making any sleep you get far less restful and rejuvenating.

- "Willing" yourself to sleep doesn't work. In fact, trying to force yourself to sleep is probably going to increase your anxiety, making it even more difficult to fall asleep. If you find that you've been lying in bed awake for more than twenty or thirty minutes, get up and do something quiet and relaxing that you can stop doing at any time, such as reading a book. Keep in mind that the goal is to return to bed as soon as you start to feel drowsy. For this reason, watching television generally isn't recommended, as some programs can be emotionally intense or can draw you in and make it even harder to get back to sleep.

- Try to avoid using electronic devices, such as computers, smartphones, or tablets, in the hour or so before your bedtime. The artificial light from these devices can trigger areas of your brain involved in wakefulness, making it more difficult to fall asleep. In addition, if these devices are connected with work, school, or interpersonal problems in your life, using them may remind you of these stressors, causing your mind to start spinning, worrying, or ruminating right before bedtime.

- Make your bedroom a relaxing and comfortable place. Keep it at a cool temperature. Consider buying noise-blocking earplugs or an eye mask to block out any outside sounds or light.

- Limit the activities you do in your bedroom. Make it about sleep and sex and nothing else. Don't watch television in your bedroom or use your computer while in bed. You want your bedroom to be associated with sleep. This can help trigger your body to start the process of falling asleep as soon as you go to bed.

As you can see, there is a lot involved in establishing and maintaining a regular sleep schedule. It's a process, and improving your sleep may take some time. Don't get discouraged if you find that the tips above aren't working right away. They will eventually, and when they do, you will notice that maintaining a regular sleep schedule is extremely beneficial for your physical and emotional well-being.

Getting Regular Exercise

Another way to improve your mental health is to exercise regularly (Linehan 1993b). Regular exercise can actually increase your body's ability to withstand stress. This doesn't mean that you necessarily have to go to a gym and work out five days a week. Although that's one good option for getting into a regular exercise routine, there are many others as well. Therefore, even if you don't have the time or money to join a gym or go to one regularly, you can still get the physical benefits of exercise.

All you need to do is some sort of moderate physical activity for thirty minutes a day, five days a week. This could mean running or lifting weights, or it could mean gardening, walking, taking the stairs instead of the elevator, or parking farther away from the store entrance when you go shopping. Exercise can come in a number of different forms. The key is simply to find an activity that gets your heart rate up. In fact, the more creative you are in coming up with activities, the better. This can make exercise seem more fun and less like a chore. It can also help you stick with a regular exercise routine even when you have a lot of other things going on in your life.

Taking Care of Illnesses

Physical illness can drain your body's resources and have a negative impact on your emotional health. Therefore, it's important to take care of any physical illnesses you have (Linehan 1993b). If you think you're coming down with something, see a doctor. If your doctor prescribes medications, make sure you take them as prescribed. Take care of yourself when you are sick. Get enough rest, even if it means sleeping more than usual or resting during the day. Eat well and make sure to get plenty of vitamins. Give yourself permission to take a day off and focus only on getting better. Taking these steps will help you recover more quickly and limit the toll your physical illness takes on your mental health.

Limiting Alcohol and Avoiding Drugs

Alcohol and drugs are mind- and mood-altering substances. They can negatively affect your sleep, appetite, and energy levels, as well as your overall emotional well-being. People often choose to use alcohol or drugs as a way of coping with emotional distress. Although doing so can provide relief in the moment, this relief is temporary. Alcohol and drugs don't address the actual problem or source of distress, and any emotions they help you escape will eventually return. What's more, when these emotions return, they may be more intense and accompanied by other emotions that weren't even there initially, such as guilt or shame. For these reasons, even though the pull to use alcohol or drugs may be strong, it's best to limit your use of alcohol and to steer clear of drugs altogether (Linehan 1993b). Doing so will keep your body functioning at its optimal level and help you maintain your emotional health.

SURROUNDING YOURSELF WITH POSITIVE RELATIONSHIPS

Another way to improve your mental health is to establish strong sources of emotional support. It would be great if you always had the resources or knowledge to deal with all of the stressful experiences that come your way. However, there will be times when you don't know how best to manage a stressful situation. At these times, getting advice, support, or guidance from someone else may be just what you need. Another person may be able to look at the problem with fresh eyes and provide you with a new perspective. That person could also just be there to listen and provide you with emotional support. Sometimes, that's all you may need to feel a little better and more capable of handling the situation.

When you are identifying possible sources of support, choose people you trust and feel comfortable being honest with. It's also a good idea to choose someone who is likely to validate your experiences. You want to be able to express your emotions without fear of being invalidated, belittled, or punished. Choosing someone who you know will usually be available to provide support when you need it is also important. Even the most trustworthy and compassionate people won't be great sources of support if they are never around or are too busy to call you back.

ENGAGING IN POSITIVE ACTIVITIES

Another way to support your mental health is to take steps to build a life that is meaningful, positive, and enriching (Hayes, Strosahl, and Wilson 1999). All too often, we get so caught up in the stress of everyday life and trying to accomplish all of our day-to-day tasks that we don't leave time for the things that bring meaning to our lives or move us forward. One way to improve your emotional well-being is to start doing things that matter to you and that are consistent with the kind of life you want to live. The skills in this section are adapted from Dr. Steve Hayes's work on acceptance and commitment therapy, a behavioral treatment that has a lot of overlap with DBT (Hayes, Strosahl, and Wilson 1999).

The first step in building a meaningful life is to think about what matters to you in life. It may be helpful to think about different areas of your life, such as romantic or family relationships, friendships, work, education, leisure activities, and religion or spirituality. Then ask yourself how important each of these areas is to you. For those that are important, think about how much time you've been devoting to them and how often you make them a priority in terms of your weekly activities. For example, you might find that leisure matters to you, but your work schedule or family or school responsibilities prevent you from taking advantage of any opportunities to engage in leisure activities. Does this sound familiar? Many of us have so many demands in our lives that it is difficult to find the time to do the things we want to do or enjoy doing. If you can relate to this, the good news is that it's never too late. You can begin correcting this problem right now!

Once you've figured out the areas of life that are most important to you, the next step is to start brainstorming different activities in these areas that you can engage in regularly. When doing this exercise, people often start coming up with big goals that they want to accomplish in these important areas. Although there's nothing wrong with coming up with some long-term goals, the point of this exercise is to identify things that you can do right away. Therefore, try to come up with some small activities that you can start doing immediately and that you can do on a regular basis. One big activity may make you feel great in the moment, but filling your week with a number of small activities that matter to you will have greater mental health benefits. These activities may be small, but they will add up and give you the chance to connect with something that is positive and meaningful every day.

You may also find it helpful to schedule specific times to do some of these activities, particularly at the beginning. Doing so may make you more likely to follow through with these activities. That said, we also encourage you to start out slow. Although we want you to start building a meaningful life for yourself, we don't want that process to become a new source of stress. For now, just come up with a handful of activities you can engage in each week and slowly build from there. You may also want to work on becoming more aware of opportunities to do things that matter to you in the course of your daily life. For example, let's say that it's important to you to help other people. If you're in line at the grocery store and notice that you have twenty items but the woman behind you only has one item, this is an opportunity to do something that matters to you. In that moment, you can choose to let the woman go ahead of you. This might seem like a small gesture, but that's not what matters; what matters is that you took control and made a choice to do something meaningful to you. Over time, these small choices will add up and have a big impact on your emotional well-being.

MOVING FORWARD

You might think that much of what we presented in this chapter is common sense: Eat well. Get enough sleep. Exercise. Do things that matter to you. However, just because these suggestions sound like no-brainers doesn't mean that they are easy to do. Developing a healthy lifestyle can take a lot of work and frequent reminders.

As you work on making these changes, be compassionate with yourself. Even though you may know that there are healthier choices you could be making with regard to your lifestyle, there may be times when life gets so busy or you become so overwhelmed with other responsibilities that you lose sight of these healthier choices. You may decide to skip a meal or stay up really late to meet a deadline. You might decide to sleep in on the weekend instead of going for that morning run. You may choose to comfort yourself at the end of a hard day with your favorite fast-food meal. That's okay. You don't need to be perfect. We don't expect you to be.

If you sometimes make choices that are not in line with the recommendations in this chapter, go easy on yourself. Don't beat yourself up; the more you do, the harder it will be to get back on track. Instead, give yourself permission to slip every now and then. If you do, you'll probably find that you actually slip less than before. The important thing is not to avoid all slips, but to notice when they happen and then recommit to getting back on track and creating as healthy a lifestyle as you can. As you do, you'll be creating a strong foundation on which to build all of the skills that will help you recover from BPD.

REFERENCES

American Psychiatric Association. 2000. *Diagnostic and Statistical Manual of Mental Disorders*, 4th ed., text revision. Washington, DC: American Psychiatric Association.

Bateman, A., and P. Fonagy. 1999. "Effectiveness of Partial Hospitalization in the Treatment of Borderline Personality Disorder: A Randomized Controlled Trial." *American Journal of Psychiatry* 156:1563–1569.

Bateman, A., and P. Fonagy. 2008. "8-Year Follow-Up of Patients Treated for Borderline Personality Disorder: Mentalization-Based Treatment versus Treatment as Usual." *American Journal of Psychiatry* 165:631–638.

Bateman, A., and P. Fonagy. 2009. "Randomized Controlled Trial of Outpatient Mentalization-Based Treatment versus Structured Clinical Management for Borderline Personality Disorder." *American Journal of Psychiatry* 166:1355–1364.

Bourne, E. 1995. *The Anxiety and Phobia Workbook*. Oakland, CA: New Harbinger Publications.

Brown, M., K. Comtois, and M. Linehan. 2002. "Reasons for Suicide Attempts and Nonsuicidal Self-Injury in Women with Borderline Personality Disorder. *Journal of Abnormal Psychology* 111:198–202.

Chapman, A., K. Gratz, and M. Brown. 2006. "Solving the Puzzle of Deliberate Self-Harm: The Experiential Avoidance Model." *Behaviour Research and Therapy* 44:371–394.

Ebner-Priemer, U., J. Kuo, W. Schlotz, N. Kleindienst, M. Rosenthal, L. Detterer, and M. Bohus. 2008. "Distress and Affective Dysregulation in Patients with Borderline Personality Disorder: A Psychophysiological Ambulatory Monitoring Study." *Journal of Nervous and Mental Disease* 196:314–320.

Frances, A., M. Fyer, and J. Clarkin. 1986. "Personality and Suicide." *Annals of the New York Academy of Science* 487:281–293.

Grant, B., S. Chou, R. Goldstein, B. Huang, F. Stinson, T. Saha, S. Smith, D. Dawson, A. Pulay, R. Pickering, and W. Ruan. 2008. "Prevalence, Correlates, Disability, and Comorbidity of

DSM-IV Borderline Personality Disorder: Results from the Wave 2 National Epidemiologic Survey on Alcohol and Related Conditions." *Journal of Clinical Psychiatry* 69:533–545.

Gratz, K., and J. Gunderson. 2006. "Preliminary Data on Acceptance-Based Emotion Regulation Group Intervention for Deliberate Self-Harm among Women with Borderline Personality Disorder." *Behavior Therapy* 37:25–35.

Gratz, K., and M. Tull. 2011. "Extending Research on the Utility of an Adjunctive Emotion Regulation Group Therapy for Deliberate Self-Harm among Women with Borderline Personality Pathology." *Personality Disorders: Theory, Research, and Treatment* 2:316–326.

Gunderson, J., with P. Links. 2001. *Borderline Personality Disorder: A Clinical Guide*. Washington, DC: American Psychiatric Association.

Hayes, S., K. Strosahl, and K. Wilson. 1999. *Acceptance and Commitment Therapy: An Experiential Approach to Behavior Change*. New York: Guilford Press.

Lieb, K., B. Vollm, G. Rucker, A. Timmer, and J. M. Stoffers. 2010. "Pharmacotherapy for Borderline Personality Disorder: Cochrane Systematic Review of Randomised Trials." *British Journal of Psychiatry* 196:4–12.

Lieb, K., M. Zanarini, C. Schmahl, M. Linehan, and M. Bohus. 2004. Borderline personality disorder. *Lancet* 364:453–461.

Lieberman, M., N. Eisenberger, M. Crockett, S. Tom, J. Pfeifer, and B. Way. 2007. "Putting Feelings into Words." *Psychological Science* 18:421–429.

Linehan, M. 1993a. *Cognitive-Behavioral Treatment of Borderline Personality Disorder.* New York: Guilford Press.

Linehan, M. 1993b. *Skills Training Manual for Treatment of Borderline Personality Disorder.* New York: Guilford Press.

Linehan, M. In press. Skills Training Manual for Disordered Emotion Regulation. New York: The Guilford Press.

Link, B., E. Struening, S. Neese-Todd, S. Asmussen, and J. Phelan. 2001. "Stigma as a Barrier to Recovery: The Consequences of Stigma for the Self-Esteem of People with Mental Illnesses." *Psychiatric Services* 52:1621–1626.

Lynch, T., J. Cheavens, K. Cukrowicz, S. Thorp, L. Bronner, and J. Beyer. 2007. "Treatment of Older Adults with Co-morbid Personality Disorder and Depression: A Dialectical Behavior Therapy Approach." *International Journal of Geriatric Psychiatry* 22:131–143.

Markowitz, F. 1998. "The Effects of Stigma on the Psychological Well-Being and Life Satisfaction of Persons with Mental Illness." *Journal of Health and Social Behavior* 39:335–347.

Perlis, M. L., C. Jungquist, M. T. Smith, and D. Posner. 2008. *Cognitive Behavioral Treatment of Insomnia: A Session-by-Session Guide.* New York: Springer.

Robins, C., and A. Chapman. 2004. "Dialectical Behavior Therapy: Current Status, Recent Developments, and Future Directions." *Journal of Personality Disorders* 18:73–89.

Ruocco, A. C., S. Amirthavasagam, L. W. Choi-Kain, and S. F. McMain. 2012. "Neural Correlates of Negative Emotionality in Borderline Personality Disorder: An Activation-Likelihood-Estimation Meta-Analysis." *Biological Psychiatry* 73(2):153–160.

Ruocco, A. C., S. Amirthavasagam, and K. K. Zakzanis. 2012. "Amygdala and Hippocampal Volume Reductions and Candidate Endophenotypes for Borderline Personality Disorder: A Meta-Analysis of Magnetic Resonance Imaging Studies." *Psychiatry Research* 201(3):245–252.

Sirey, J., M. Bruce, G. Alexopoulos, D. Perlick, S. Friedman, and B. Meyers. 2001. "Stigma as a Barrier to Recovery: Perceived Stigma and Patient-Rated Severity of Illness as Predictors of Antidepressant Drug Adherence." *Psychiatric Services* 52:1615–1620.

Stoffers, J., B. Völlm, G. Rücker, A. Timmer, N. Huband, and K. Lieb. 2010. "Pharmacological Interventions for Borderline Personality Disorder." *Cochrane Database of Systematic Reviews* 6:CD005653.

Torgersen, S. 2000. "Genetics of Patients with Borderline Personality Disorder." *Psychiatric Clinics of North America* 23:1–9.

Zanarini, M. 2000. "Childhood Experiences Associated with the Development of Borderline Personality Disorder." *Psychiatric Clinics of North America* 23(1):89–101.

Zanarini, M., F. Frankenburg, D. Reich, and G. Fitzmaurice. 2010. "The 10-Year Course of Psychosocial Functioning among Patients with Borderline Personality Disorder and Axis II Comparison Subjects." *Acta Psychiatrica Scandinavica* 122:103–109.

Zanarini, M., J. Gunderson, M. Marino, and E. Schwartz. 1988. "*DSM-III* Disorders in the Families of Borderline Outpatients." *Journal of Personality Disorders* 2:292–302.

Zanarini, M., L. Yong, F. Frankenburg, J. Hennen, D. Reich, M. Marino, and A. Vujanovic. 2002. "Severity of Reported Childhood Sexual Abuse and Its Relationship to Severity of Borderline Psychopathology and Psychosocial Impairment among Borderline Inpatients." *Journal of Nervous and Mental Disease* 190:381–387.

Zimmerman, D. J., and L. W. Choi-Kain. 2009. "The Hypothalamic-Pituitary-Adrenal Axis in Borderline Personality Disorder: A Review." *Harvard Review of Psychiatry* 17(3):167–183.

Alexander L. Chapman, PhD, RPsych, is a registered psychologist and an associate professor in the department of psychology at Simon Fraser University, as well as the president of the DBT Centre of Vancouver. Chapman directs the personality and emotion research laboratory, where he studies the role of emotion regulation in borderline personality disorder (BPD), self-harm, impulsivity, and other behavioral problems. His research is funded by the Canadian Institutes of Health Research and the Social Sciences and Humanities Research Council of Canada. Chapman received the Young Investigator Award of the National Education Alliance for BPD (2007), the Canadian Psychological Association's (CPA) Scientist Practitioner Early Career Award, and a Career Investigator award from the Michael Smith Foundation for Health Research. He has coauthored five books, three of which received the 2012 Association for Behavioral and Cognitive Therapies Self-Help Book Seal of Merit Award.

Kim L. Gratz, PhD, is an associate professor in the department of psychiatry and human behavior at the University of Mississippi Medical Center, where she serves as director of personality disorders research and director of the dialectical behavior therapy (DBT) clinic. In 2005, Gratz received the Young Investigator Award of the National Education Alliance for BPD. Gratz has written numerous journal articles and book chapters on borderline personality disorder, deliberate self-harm, and emotion regulation (among other topics), and is coauthor of several books, including *The Borderline Personality Disorder Survival Guide, Freedom from Self-Harm*, and *The Dialectical Behavior Therapy Skills Workbook for Anxiety*. Gratz currently serves as principal investigator or co-investigator on several major grants from the National Institutes of Health.

MORE BOOKS *from*
NEW HARBINGER PUBLICATIONS

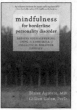

MINDFULNESS FOR BORDERLINE PERSONALITY DISORDER
Relieve Your Suffering Using the Core Skill of Dialectical Behavior Therapy
ISBN: 978-1608825653
US $16.95
Also available as an e-book

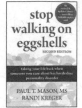

STOP WALKING ON EGGSHELLS, SECOND EDITION
Taking Your Life Back When Someone You Care About Has Borderline Personality Disorder
ISBN: 978-1572246904
US $18.95
Also available as an e-book

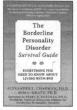

BORDERLINE PERSONALITY DISORDER SURVIVAL GUIDE
Everything You Need to Know About Living with BPD
ISBN: 978-1572245075
US $16.95
Also available as an e-book

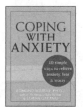

COPING WITH ANXIETY
10 Simple Ways to Relieve Anxiety, Fear & Worry
ISBN: 978-1572243200
US $14.95
Also available as an e-book

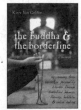

THE BUDDHA & THE BORDERLINE
My Recovery from Borderline Personality Disorder through Dialectical Behavior Therapy, Buddhism & Online Dating
ISBN: 978-1572247109
US $17.95
Also available as an e-book

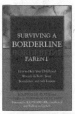

SURVIVING A BORDERLINE PARENT
How to Heal Your Childhood Wounds & Build Trust, Boundaries & Self-Esteem
ISBN: 978-1572243286
US $16.95
Also available as an e-book

new harbinger publications, inc.
1-800-748-6273 / newharbinger.com

(VISA, MC, AMEX / prices subject to change without notice)

Like us on Facebook   Follow us on Twitter @newharbinger.com

Don't miss out on new books in the subjects that interest you.
Sign up for our **Book Alerts** at **newharbinger.com/bookalerts**

FROM OUR PUBLISHER—

As the publisher at New Harbinger and a clinical psychologist since 1978, I know that emotional problems are best helped with evidence-based therapies. These are the treatments derived from scientific research (randomized controlled trials) that show what works. Whether these treatments are delivered by trained clinicians or found in a self-help book, they are designed to provide you with proven strategies to overcome your problem.

Therapies that aren't evidence-based—whether offered by clinicians or in books—are much less likely to help. In fact, therapies that aren't guided by science may not help you at all. That's why this New Harbinger book is based on scientific evidence that the treatment can relieve emotional pain.

This is important: if this book isn't enough, and you need the help of a skilled therapist, use the following resources to find a clinician trained in the evidence-based protocols appropriate for your problem. And if you need more support—a community that understands what you're going through and can show you ways to cope—resources for that are provided below, as well.

Real help is available for the problems you have been struggling with. The skills you can learn from evidence-based therapies will change your life.

new harbinger
CELEBRATING
40 YEARS

Matthew McKay, PhD
Publisher, New Harbinger Publications

If you need a therapist, the following organization can help you find a therapist trained in dialectical behavior therapy (DBT).

Behavioral Tech, LLC

Please visit www.behavioraltech.org and click on *Find a DBT Therapist*.

For support for patients, family, and friends, please contact the following:

BPD Central

Visit www.bpdcentral.org

Treatment and Research Advancements Association for Personality Disorder (TARA)

Visit www.tara4bpd.org

National Suicide Prevention Lifeline

Call 24 hours a day 1-800-273-TALK (8255) or visit suicidepreventionlifeline.org

For more new harbinger books, visit www.newharbinger.com

Register your **new harbinger** titles for additional benefits!

When you register your **new harbinger** title—purchased in any format, from any source—you get access to benefits like the following:

- Downloadable accessories like printable worksheets and extra content
- Instructional videos and audio files
- Information about updates, corrections, and new editions

Not every title has accessories, but we're adding new material all the time.

Access free accessories in 3 easy steps:

1. Sign in at NewHarbinger.com (or **register** to create an account).

2. Click on **register a book**. Search for your title and click the **register** button when it appears.

3. Click on the **book cover or title** to go to its details page. Click on **accessories** to view and access files.

That's all there is to it!

If you need help, visit:

NewHarbinger.com/accessories

new harbinger
CELEBRATING
40 YEARS

31901055197851